DASH RECIPES

2022

LOW SODIUM DELICIOUS RECIPES TO LOWER BLOOD

PRESSURE

OLIVIA SPEED

Table of Contents

Mustard Greens Sauté

Preparation time: 10 minutes
Cooking time: 12 minutes
Servings: 4

Ingredients:
- 6 cups mustard greens
- 2 tablespoons olive oil
- 2 spring onions, chopped
- ½ cup coconut cream
- 2 tablespoons sweet paprika
- Black pepper to the taste

Directions:
1. Heat up a pan with the oil over medium-high heat, add the onions, paprika and black pepper, stir and sauté for 3 minutes.
2. Add the mustard greens and the other ingredients, toss, cook for 9 minutes more, divide between plates and serve as a side dish.

Nutrition: calories 163, fat 14.8, fiber 4.9, carbs 8.3, protein 3.6

Bok Choy Mix

Preparation time: 10 minutes
Cooking time: 12 minutes
Servings: 4

Ingredients:

- 1 tablespoon avocado oil
- 1 tablespoon balsamic vinegar
- 1 yellow onion, chopped
- 1 pound bok choy, torn
- 1 teaspoon cumin, ground
- 1 tablespoon coconut aminos
- ¼ cup low-sodium veggie stock
- Black pepper to the taste

Directions:

1. Heat up a pan with the oil over medium-high heat, add the onion, cumin and black pepper, stir and cook for 3 minutes.
2. Add the bok choy and the other ingredients, toss, cook for 8-9 minutes more, divide between plates and serve as a side dish.

Nutrition: calories 38, fat 0.8, fiber 2, carbs 6.5, protein 2.2

Green Beans and Eggplant Mix

Preparation time: 4 minutes
Cooking time: 40 minutes
Servings: 4

Ingredients:
- 1 pound green beans, trimmed and halved
- 1 small eggplant, cut into large chunks
- 1 yellow onion, chopped
- 2 tablespoons olive oil
- 2 tablespoons lime juice
- 1 teaspoon smoked paprika
- ¼ cup low-sodium veggie stock
- Black pepper to the taste
- ½ teaspoon oregano, dried

Directions:
1. In a roasting pan, combine the green beans with the eggplant and the other ingredients, toss, introduce in the oven, bake at 390 degrees F for 40 minutes, divide between plates and serve as a side dish.

Nutrition: calories 141, fat 7.5, fiber 8.9, carbs 19, protein 3.7

Olives and Artichokes Mix

Preparation time: 5 minutes
Cooing time: 0 minutes
Servings: 4

Ingredients:

- 10 ounces canned artichoke hearts, no-salt-added, drained and halved
- 1 cup black olives, pitted and sliced
- 1 tablespoon capers, drained
- 1 cup green olives, pitted and sliced
- 1 tablespoon parsley, chopped
- Black pepper to the taste
- 2 tablespoons olive oil
- 2 tablespoons red wine vinegar
- 1 tablespoon chives, chopped

Directions:

1. In a salad bowl, combine the artichokes with the olives and the other ingredients, toss and serve as a side dish.

Nutrition: calories 138, fat 11, fiber 5.1, carbs 10, protein 2.7

Turmeric Peppers Dip

Preparation time: 4 minutes
Cooking time: 0 minutes
Servings: 4

Ingredients:
- 1 teaspoon turmeric powder
- 1 cup coconut cream
- 14 ounces red peppers, no-salt-added, chopped
- Juice of ½ lemon
- 1 tablespoon chives, chopped

Directions:
1. In your blender, combine the peppers with the turmeric and the other ingredients except the chives, pulse well, divide into bowls and serve as a snack with the chives sprinkled on top.

Nutrition: calories 183, fat 14.9, fiber 3. carbs 12.7, protein 3.4

Lentils Spread

Preparation time: 5 minutes
Cooking time: 0 minutes
Servings: 4

Ingredients:

- 14 ounces canned lentils, drained, no-salt-added, rinsed
- Juice of 1 lemon
- 2 garlic cloves, minced
- 2 tablespoons olive oil
- ½ cup cilantro, chopped

Directions:

1. In a blender, combine the lentils with the oil and the other ingredients, pulse well, divide into bowls and serve as a party spread.

Nutrition: calories 416, fat 8.2, fiber 30.4, carbs 60.4, protein 25.8

Roasted Walnuts

Preparation time: 5 minutes
Cooking time: 15 minutes
Servings: 8

Ingredients:
- ½ teaspoon smoked paprika
- ½ teaspoon chili powder
- ½ teaspoon garlic powder
- 1 tablespoon avocado oil
- A pinch of cayenne pepper
- 14 ounces walnuts

Directions:
1. Spread the walnuts on a lined baking sheet, add the paprika and the other ingredients, toss and bake at 410 degrees F for 15 minutes.
2. Divide into bowls and serve as a snack.

Nutrition: calories 311, fat 29.6, fiber 3.6, carbs 5.3, protein 12

Cranberry Squares

Preparation time: 3 hours and 5 minutes

Cooking time: 0 minutes
Servings: 4

Ingredients:
- 2 ounces coconut cream
- 2 tablespoons rolled oats
- 2 tablespoons coconut, shredded
- 1 cup cranberries

Directions:
1. In a blender, combine the oats with the cranberries and the other ingredients, pulse well and spread into a square pan.

Cut into squares and keep them in the fridge for 3 hours before serving.

Nutrition: calories 66, fat 4.4, fiber 1.8, carbs 5.4, protein 0.8

Cauliflower Bars

Preparation time: 10 minutes
Cooking time: 30 minutes
Servings: 8

Ingredients:
- 2 cups whole wheat flour
- 2 teaspoons baking powder
- A pinch of black pepper
- 2 eggs, whisked
- 1 cup almond milk
- 1 cup cauliflower florets, chopped
- ½ cup low-fat cheddar, shredded

Directions:
1. In a bowl, combine the flour with the cauliflower and the other ingredients and stir well.
2. Spread into a baking tray, introduce in the oven, bake at 400 degrees F for 30 minutes, cut into bars and serve as a snack.

Nutrition: calories 430, fat 18.1, fiber 3.7, carbs 54, protein 14.5

Almonds and Seeds Bowls

Preparation time: 5 minutes
Cooking time: 10 minutes
Servings: 4

Ingredients:

- 2 cups almonds
- ¼ cup coconut, shredded
- 1 mango, peeled and cubed
- 1 cup sunflower seeds
- Cooking spray

Directions:

1. Spread the almonds, coconut, mango and sunflower seeds on a baking tray, grease with the cooking spray, toss and bake at 400 degrees F for 10 minutes.
2. Divide into bowls and serve as a snack.

Nutrition: calories 411, fat 31.8, fiber 8.7, carbs 25.8, protein 13.3

Potato Chips

Preparation time: 10 minutes
Cooking time: 20 minutes
Servings: 4

Ingredients:

- 4 gold potatoes, peeled and thinly sliced
- 2 tablespoons olive oil
- 1 tablespoon chili powder
- 1 teaspoon sweet paprika
- 1 tablespoon chives, chopped

Directions:

1. Spread the chips on a lined baking sheet, add the oil and the other ingredients, toss, introduce in the oven and bake at 390 degrees F for 20 minutes.
2. Divide into bowls and serve.

Nutrition: calories 118, fat 7.4, fiber 2.9, carbs 13.4, protein 1.3

Kale Dip

Preparation time: 10 minutes
Cooking time: 20 minutes
Servings: 4

Ingredients:
- 1 bunch kale leaves
- 1 cup coconut cream
- 1 shallot, chopped
- 1 tablespoon olive oil
- 1 teaspoon chili powder
- A pinch of black pepper

Directions:
1. Heat up a pan with the oil over medium heat, add the shallots, stir and sauté for 4 minutes.
2. Add the kale and the other ingredients, bring to a simmer and cook over medium heat for 16 minutes.
3. Blend using an immersion blender, divide into bowls and serve as a snack.

Nutrition: calories 188, fat 17.9, fiber 2.1, carbs 7.6, protein 2.5

Beets Chips

Preparation time: 10 minutes
Cooking time: 35 minutes
Servings: 4

Ingredients:

- 2 beets, peeled and thinly sliced
- 1 tablespoon avocado oil
- 1 teaspoon cumin, ground
- 1 teaspoon fennel seeds, crushed
- 2 teaspoons garlic, minced

Directions:

1. Spread the beet chips on a lined baking sheet, add the oil and the other ingredients, toss, introduce in the oven and bake at 400 degrees F for 35 minutes.
2. Divide into bowls and serve as a snack.

Nutrition: calories 32, fat 0.7, fiber 1.4, carbs 6.1, protein 1.1

Zucchini Dip

Preparation time: 5 minutes
Cooking time: 10 minutes
Servings: 4

Ingredients:

- ½ cup nonfat yogurt
- 2 zucchinis, chopped
- 1 tablespoon olive oil
- 2 spring onions, chopped
- ¼ cup low-sodium veggie stock
- 2 garlic cloves, minced
- 1 tablespoon dill, chopped
- A pinch of nutmeg, ground

Directions:

1. Heat up a pan with the oil over medium heat, add the onions and garlic, stir and sauté for 3 minutes.
2. Add the zucchinis and the other ingredients except the yogurt, toss, cook for 7 minutes more and take off the heat.
3. Add the yogurt, blend using an immersion blender, divide into bowls and serve.

Nutrition: calories 76, fat 4.1, fiber 1.5, carbs 7.2, protein 3.4

Seeds and Apple Mix

Preparation time: 10 minutes
Cooking time: 20 minutes
Servings: 4

Ingredients:

- 2 tablespoons olive oil
- 1 teaspoon smoked paprika
- 1 cup sunflower seeds
- 1 cup chia seeds
- 2 apples, cored and cut into wedges
- ½ teaspoon cumin, ground
- A pinch of cayenne pepper

Directions:

1. In a bowl, combine the seeds with the apples and the other ingredients, toss, spread on a lined baking sheet, introduce in the oven and bake at 350 degrees F for 20 minutes.
2. Divide into bowls and serve as a snack.

Nutrition: calories 222, fat 15.4, fiber 6.4, carbs 21.1, protein 4

Pumpkin Spread

Preparation time: 5 minutes
Cooking time: 0 minutes
Servings: 4

Ingredients:
- 2 cups pumpkin flesh
- ½ cup pumpkin seeds
- 1 tablespoon lemon juice
- 1 tablespoon sesame seed paste
- 1 tablespoon olive oil

Directions:
1. In a blender, combine the pumpkin with the seeds and the other ingredients, pulse well, divide into bowls and serve a party spread.

Nutrition: calories 162, fat 12.7, fiber 2.3, carbs 9.7, protein 5.5

Spinach Spread

Preparation time: 10 minutes
Cooking time: 20 minutes
Servings: 4

Ingredients:
- 1 pound spinach, chopped
- 1 cup coconut cream
- 1 cup low-fat mozzarella, shredded
- A pinch of black pepper
- 1 tablespoon dill, chopped

Directions:
1. In a baking pan, combine the spinach with the cream and the other ingredients, stir well, introduce in the oven and bake at 400 degrees F for 20 minutes.
2. Divide into bowls and serve.

Nutrition: calories 186, fat 14.8, fiber 4.4, carbs 8.4, protein 8.8

Olives and Cilantro Salsa

Preparation time: 5 minutes
Cooking time: 0 minutes
Servings: 4

Ingredients:
- 1 red onion, chopped
- 1 cup black olives, pitted and halved
- 1 cucumber, cubed
- ¼ cup cilantro, chopped
- A pinch of black pepper
- 2 tablespoons lime juice

Directions:
1. In a bowl, combine the olives with the cucumber and the rest of the ingredients, toss and serve cold as a snack.

Nutrition: calories 64, fat 3.7, fiber 2.1, carbs 8.4, protein 1.1

Chives and Beets Dip

Preparation time: 5 minutes
Cooking time: 25 minutes
Servings: 4

Ingredients:

- 2 tablespoons olive oil
- 1 red onion, chopped
- 2 tablespoons chives, chopped
- A pinch of black pepper
- 1 beet, peeled and chopped
- 8 ounces low-fat cream cheese
- 1 cup coconut cream

Directions:

1. Heat up a pan with the oil over medium heat, add the onion and sauté for 5 minutes.
2. Add the rest of the ingredients, and cook everything for 20 minutes more stirring often.
3. Transfer the mix to a blender, pulse well, divide into bowls and serve.

Nutrition: calories 418, fat 41.2, fiber 2.5, carbs 10, protein 6.4

Cucumber Salsa

Preparation time: 5 minutes
Cooking time: 0 minutes
Servings: 4

Ingredients:
- 1 pound cucumbers cubed
- 1 avocado, peeled, pitted and cubed
- 1 tablespoon capers, drained
- 1 tablespoon chives, chopped
- 1 small red onion, cubed
- 1 tablespoon olive oil
- 1 tablespoon balsamic vinegar

Directions:
1. In a bowl, combine the cucumbers with the avocado and the other ingredients, toss, divide into small cups and serve.

Nutrition: calories 132, fat 4.4, fiber 4, carbs 11.6, protein 4.5

Chickpeas Dip

Preparation time: 5 minutes
Cooking time: 0 minutes
Servings: 4

Ingredients:
- 1 tablespoon olive oil
- 1 tablespoon lemon juice
- 1 tablespoon sesame seeds paste
- 2 tablespoons chives, chopped
- 2 spring onions, chopped
- 2 cups canned chickpeas, no-salt-added, drained and rinsed

Directions:
1. In your blender, combine the chickpeas with the oil and the other ingredients except the chives, pulse well, divide into bowls, sprinkle the chives on top and serve.

Nutrition: calories 280, fat 13.3, fiber 5.5, carbs 14.8, protein 6.2

Olives Dip

Preparation time: 4 minutes
Cooking time: 0 minutes
Servings: 4

Ingredients:
- 2 cups black olives, pitted and chopped
- 1 cup mint, chopped
- 2 tablespoons avocado oil
- ½ cup coconut cream
- ¼ cup lime juice
- A pinch of black pepper

Directions:
1. In your blender, combine the olives with the mint and the other ingredients, pulse well, divide into bowls and serve.

Nutrition: calories 287, fat 13.3, fiber 4.7, carbs 17.4, protein 2.4

Coconut Onions Dip

Preparation time: 5 minutes
Cooking time: 0 minutes
Servings: 4

Ingredients:
- 4 spring onions, chopped
- 1 shallot, minced
- 1 tablespoon lime juice
- A pinch of black pepper
- 2 ounces low-fat mozzarella cheese, shredded
- 1 cup coconut cream
- 1 tablespoon parsley, chopped

Directions:
1. In a blender, combine the spring onions with the shallot and the other ingredients, pulse well, divide into bowls and serve as a party dip.

Nutrition: calories 271, fat 15.3, fiber 5, carbs 15.9, protein 6.9

Pine Nuts and Coconut Dip

Preparation time: 5 minutes
Cooking time: 0 minutes
Servings: 4

Ingredients:

- 8 ounces coconut cream
- 1 tablespoon pine nuts, chopped
- 2 tablespoons parsley, chopped
- A pinch of black pepper

Directions:

1. In a bowl, combine the cream with the pine nuts and the rest of the ingredients, whisk well, divide into bowls and serve.

Nutrition: calories 281, fat 13, fiber 4.8, carbs 16, protein 3.56

Arugula and Cucumbers Salsa

Preparation time: 5 minutes
Cooking time: 0 minutes
Servings: 4

Ingredients:

- 4 scallions, chopped
- 2 tomatoes, cubed
- 4 cucumbers, cubed
- 1 tablespoon balsamic vinegar
- 1 cup baby arugula leaves
- 2 tablespoons lemon juice
- 2 tablespoons olive oil
- A pinch of black pepper

Directions:

1. In a bowl, combine the scallions with the tomatoes and the other ingredients, toss, divide into small bowls and serve as a snack.

Nutrition: calories 139, fat 3.8, fiber 4.5, carbs 14, protein 5.4

Cheese Dip

Preparation time: 5 minutes
Cooking time: 0 minutes
Servings: 6

Ingredients:
- 1 tablespoon mint, chopped
- 1 tablespoon oregano, chopped
- 10 ounces non-fat cream cheese
- ½ cup ginger, sliced
- 2 tablespoons coconut aminos

Directions:
1. In your blender, combine the cream cheese with the ginger and the other ingredients, pulse well, divide into small cups and serve.

Nutrition: calories 388, fat 15.4, fiber 6, carbs 14.3, protein 6

Paprika Yogurt Dip

Preparation time: 5 minutes
Cooking time: 0 minutes
Servings: 4

Ingredients:
- 3 cups non-fat yogurt
- 2 spring onions, chopped
- 1 teaspoon sweet paprika
- ¼ cup almonds, chopped
- ¼ cup dill, chopped

Directions:
1. In a bowl, combine the yogurt with the onions and the other ingredients, whisk, divide into bowls and serve.

Nutrition: calories 181, fat 12.2, fiber 6, carbs 14,1, protein 7

Cauliflower Salsa

Preparation time: 5 minutes
Cooking time: 0 minutes
Servings: 4

Ingredients:
- 1 pound cauliflower florets, blanched
- 1 cup kalamata olives, pitted and halved
- 1 cup cherry tomatoes, halved
- 1 tablespoon olive oil
- 1 tablespoon lime juice
- A pinch of black pepper

Directions:
1. In a bowl, combine the cauliflower with the olives and the other ingredients, toss and serve.

Nutrition: calories 139, fat 4, fiber 3.6, carbs 5.5, protein 3.4

Shrimp Spread

Preparation time: 5 minutes
Cooking time: 0 minutes
Servings: 4

Ingredients:
- 8 ounces coconut cream
- 1 pound shrimp, cooked, peeled, deveined and chopped
- 2 tablespoons dill, chopped
- 2 spring onions, chopped
- 1 tablespoon cilantro, chopped
- A pinch of black pepper

Directions:
1. In a bowl, combine the shrimp with the cream and the other ingredients, whisk and serve as a party spread.

Nutrition: calories 362, fat 14.3, fiber 6, carbs 14.6, protein 5.9

Peach Salsa

Preparation time: 4 minutes
Cooking time: 0 minutes
Servings: 4

Ingredients:

- 4 peaches, stones removed and cubed
- 1 cup kalamata olives, pitted and halved
- 1 avocado, pitted, peeled and cubed
- 1 cup cherry tomatoes, halved
- 1 tablespoon olive oil
- 1 tablespoon lime juice
- 1 tablespoon cilantro, chopped

Directions:

1. In a bowl, combine the peaches with the olives and the other ingredients, toss well and serve cold.

Nutrition: calories 200, fat 7.5, fiber 5, carbs 13.3, protein 4.9

Carrot Chips

Preparation time: 10 minutes
Cooking time: 20 minutes
Servings: 4

Ingredients:
- 4 carrots, thinly sliced
- 2 tablespoons olive oil
- A pinch of black pepper
- 1 teaspoon sweet paprika
- ½ teaspoon turmeric powder
- A pinch of red pepper flakes

Directions:
1. In a bowl, combine the carrot chips with the oil and the other ingredients and toss.
2. Spread the chips on a lined baking sheet, bake at 400 degrees F for 25 minutes, divide into bowls and serve as a snack.

Nutrition: calories 180, fat 3, fiber 3.3, carbs 5.8, protein 1.3

Asparagus Bites

Preparation time: 4 minutes
Cooking time: 20 minutes
Servings: 4

Ingredients:
- 2 tablespoons coconut oil, melted
- 1 pound asparagus, trimmed and halved
- 1 teaspoon garlic powder
- 1 teaspoon rosemary, dried
- 1 teaspoon chili powder

Directions:
1. In a bowl, mix the asparagus with the oil and the other ingredients, toss, spread on a lined baking sheet and bake at 400 degrees F for 20 minutes.
2. Divide into bowls and serve cold as a snack.

Nutrition: calories 170, fat 4.3, fiber 4, carbs 7, protein 4.5

Baked Figs Bowls

Preparation time: 4 minutes
Cooking time: 12 minutes
Servings: 4

Ingredients:
- 8 figs, halved
- 1 tablespoon avocado oil
- 1 teaspoon nutmeg, ground

Directions:
1. In a roasting pan combine the figs with the oil and the nutmeg, toss, and bake at 400 degrees F for 12 minutes.
2. Divide the figs into small bowls and serve as a snack.

Nutrition: calories 180, fat 4.3, fiber 2, carbs 2, protein 3.2

Cabbage and Shrimp Salsa

Preparation time: 5 minutes
Cooking time: 6 minutes
Servings: 4

Ingredients:
- 2 cups red cabbage, shredded
- 1 pound shrimp, peeled and deveined
- 1 tablespoon olive oil
- A pinch of black pepper
- 2 spring onions, chopped
- 1 cup tomatoes, cubed
- ½ teaspoon garlic powder

Directions:
1. Heat up a pan with the oil over medium heat, add the shrimp, toss and cook for 3 minutes on each side.
2. In a bowl, combine the cabbage with the shrimp and the other ingredients, toss, divide into small bowls and serve.

Nutrition: calories 225, fat 9.7, fiber 5.1, carbs 11.4, protein 4.5

Avocado Wedges

Preparation time: 5 minutes
Cooking time: 10 minutes
Servings: 4

Ingredients:
- 2 avocados, peeled, pitted and cut into wedges
- 1 tablespoon avocado oil
- 1 tablespoon lime juice
- 1 teaspoon coriander, ground

Directions:
1. Spread the avocado wedges on a lined baking sheet, add the oil and the other ingredients, toss, and bake at 300 degrees F for 10 minutes.
2. Divide into cups and serve as a snack.

Nutrition: calories 212, fat 20.1, fiber 6.9, carbs 9.8, protein 2

Lemon Dip

Preparation time: 4 minutes
Cooking time: 0 minutes
Servings: 4

Ingredients:
- 1 cup low-fat cream cheese
- Black pepper to the taste
- ½ cup lemon juice
- 1 tablespoon cilantro, chopped
- 3 garlic cloves, chopped

Directions:
1. In your food processor, mix the cream cheese with the lemon juice and the other ingredients, pulse well, divide into bowls and serve.

Nutrition: calories 213, fat 20.5, fiber 0.2, carbs 2.8, protein 4.8

Sweet Potato Dip

Preparation time: 10 minutes
Cooking time: 40 minutes
Servings: 4

Ingredients:
- 1 cup sweet potatoes, peeled and cubed
- 1 tablespoon low-sodium veggie stock
- Cooking spray
- 2 tablespoons coconut cream
- 2 teaspoons rosemary, dried
- Black pepper to the taste

Directions:
1. In a baking pan, combine the potatoes with the stock and the other ingredients, stir, bake at 365 degrees F for 40 minutes, transfer to your blender, pulse well, divide into small bowls and serve

Nutrition: calories 65, fat 2.1, fiber 2, carbs 11.3, protein 0.8

Beans Salsa

Preparation time: 5 minutes
Cooking time: 0 minutes
Servings: 4

Ingredients:
- 1 cup canned black beans, no-salt-added, drained
- 1 cup canned red kidney beans, no-salt-added, drained
- 1 teaspoon balsamic vinegar
- 1 cup cherry tomatoes, cubed
- 1 tablespoon olive oil
- 2 shallots, chopped

Directions:
1. In a bowl, combine the beans with the vinegar and the other ingredients, toss and serve as a party snack.

Nutrition: calories 362, fat 4.8, fiber 14.9, carbs 61, protein 21.4

Green Beans Salsa

Preparation time: 10 minutes
Cooking time: 10 minutes
Servings: 4

Ingredients:

- 1 pound green beans, trimmed and halved
- 1 tablespoon olive oil
- 2 teaspoons capers, drained
- 6 ounces green olives, pitted and sliced
- 4 garlic cloves, minced
- 1 tablespoon lime juice
- 1 tablespoon oregano, chopped
- Black pepper to the taste

Directions:

1. Heat up a pan with the oil over medium-high heat, add the garlic and the green beans, toss and cook for 3 minutes.
2. Add the rest of the ingredients, toss, cook for another 7 minutes, divide into small cups and serve cold.

Nutrition: calories 111, fat 6.7, fiber 5.6, carbs 13.2, protein 2.9

Carrot Spread

Preparation time: 10 minutes
Cooking time: 30 minutes
Servings: 4

Ingredients:
- 1 pound carrots, peeled and chopped
- ½ cup walnuts, chopped
- 2 cups low-sodium veggie stock
- 1 cup coconut cream
- 1 tablespoon rosemary, chopped
- 1 teaspoon garlic powder
- ¼ teaspoon smoked paprika

Directions:
1. In a small pot, mix the carrots with the stock, walnuts and the other ingredients except the cream and the rosemary, stir, bring to a boil over medium heat, cook for 30 minutes, drain and transfer to a blender.
2. Add the cream, blend the mix well, divide into bowls, sprinkle the rosemary on top and serve.

Nutrition: calories 201, fat 8.7, fiber 3.4, carbs 7.8, protein 7.7

Tomato Dip

Preparation time: 10 minutes
Cooking time: 10 minutes
Servings: 4

Ingredients:
- 1 pound tomatoes, peeled and chopped
- ½ cup garlic, minced
- 2 tablespoons olive oil
- A pinch of black pepper
- 2 shallots, chopped
- 1 teaspoon thyme, dried

Directions:
1. Heat up a pan with the oil over medium-high heat, add the garlic and the shallots, stir and sauté for 2 minutes.
2. Add the tomatoes and the other ingredients, cook for 8 minutes more and transfer to a blender.
3. Pulse well, divide into small cups and serve as a snack.

Nutrition: calories 232, fat 11.3, fiber 3.9, carbs 7.9, protein 4.5

Salmon Bowls

Preparation time: 10 minutes
Cooking time: 0 minutes
Servings: 6

Ingredients:

- 1 tablespoon avocado oil
- 1 tablespoon balsamic vinegar
- ½ teaspoon oregano, dried
- 1 cup smoked salmon, no-salt-added, boneless, skinless and cubed
- 1 cup salsa
- 4 cups baby spinach

Directions:

1. In a bowl, combine the salmon with the salsa and the other ingredients, toss, divide into small cups and serve.

Nutrition: calories 281, fat 14.4, fiber 7.4, carbs 18.7, protein 7.4

Tomato and Corn Salsa

Preparation time: 4 minutes
Cooking time: 0 minutes
Servings: 4

Ingredients:
- 3 cups corn
- 2 cups tomatoes, cubed
- 2 green onions, chopped
- 2 tablespoons olive oil
- 1 red chili pepper, chopped
- ½ tablespoon chives, chopped

Directions:
1. In a salad bowl, combine the tomatoes with the corn and the other ingredients, toss and serve cold as a snack.

Nutrition: calories 178, fat 8.6, fiber 4.5, carbs 25.9, protein 4.7

Baked Mushrooms

Preparation time: 10 minutes
Cooking time: 25 minutes
Servings: 4

Ingredients:
- 1 pound small mushroom caps
- 2 tablespoons olive oil
- 1 tablespoon chives, chopped
- 1 tablespoon rosemary, chopped
- Black pepper to the taste

Directions:
1. Put the mushrooms in a roasting pan, add the oil and the rest of the ingredients, toss, bake at 400 degrees F for 25 minutes, divide into bowls and serve as a snack.

Nutrition: calories 215, fat 12.3, fiber 6.7, carbs 15.3, protein 3.5

Beans Spread

Preparation time: 5 minutes
Cooking time: 0 minutes
Servings: 4

Ingredients:
- ½ cup coconut cream
- 1 tablespoon olive oil
- 2 cups canned black beans, no-salt-added, drained and rinsed
- 2 tablespoons green onions, chopped

Directions:
1. In a blender, combine the beans with the cream and the other ingredients, pulse well, divide into bowls and serve.

Nutrition: calories 311, fat 13.5, fiber 6, carbs 18.0, protein 8

Coriander Fennel Salsa

Preparation time: 5 minutes
Cooking time: 0 minutes
Servings: 4

Ingredients:
- 2 spring onion, chopped
- 2 fennel bulbs, shredded
- 1 green chili pepper, chopped
- 1 tomato, chopped
- 1 teaspoon turmeric powder
- 1 teaspoon lime juice
- 2 tablespoons coriander, chopped
- Black pepper to the taste

Directions:
1. In a salad bowl, mix the fennel with the onions and the other ingredients, toss, divide into cups and serve.

Nutrition: calories 310, fat 11.5, fiber 5.1, carbs 22.3, protein 6.5

Brussels Sprouts Bites

Preparation time: 10 minutes
Cooking time: 25 minutes
Servings: 4

Ingredients:
- 1 pound Brussels sprouts, trimmed and halved
- 2 tablespoons olive oil
- 1 tablespoon cumin, ground
- 1 cup dill, chopped
- 2 garlic cloves, minced

Directions:
1. In a roasting pan, combine the Brussels sprouts with the oil and the other ingredients, toss and bake at 390 degrees F for 25 minutes.
2. Divide the sprouts into bowls and serve as a snack.

Nutrition: calories 270, fat 10.3, fiber 5.2, carbs 11.1, protein 6

Balsamic Walnuts Bites

Preparation time: 10 minutes
Cooking time: 15 minutes
Servings: 4

Ingredients:
- 2 cups walnuts
- 3 tablespoons red vinegar
- A drizzle of olive oil
- A pinch of cayenne pepper
- A pinch of red pepper flakes
- Black pepper to the taste

Directions:
1. Spread the walnuts on a lined baking sheet, add the vinegar and the other ingredients, toss, and roast at 400 degrees F for 15 minutes.
2. Divide the walnuts into bowls and serve.

Nutrition: calories 280, fat 12.2, fiber 2, carbs 15.8, protein 6

Radish Chips

Preparation time: 10 minutes
Cooking time: 20 minutes
Servings: 4

Ingredients:
- 1 pound radishes, thinly sliced
- A pinch of turmeric powder
- Black pepper to the taste
- 2 tablespoons olive oil

Directions:
1. Spread the radish chips on a lined baking sheet, add the oil and the other ingredients, toss and bake at 400 degrees F for 20 minutes.
2. Divide the chips into bowls and serve.

Nutrition: calories 120, fat 8.3, fiber 1, carbs 3.8, protein 6

Leeks and Shrimp Salad

Preparation time: 4 minutes
Cooking time: 0 minutes
Servings: 4

Ingredients:
- 2 leeks, sliced
- 1 cup cilantro, chopped
- 1 pound shrimp, peeled, deveined and cooked
- Juice of 1 lime
- 1 tablespoon lime zest, grated
- 1 cup cherry tomatoes, halved
- 2 tablespoons olive oil
- Salt and black pepper to the taste

Directions:
1. In a salad bowl, mix the shrimp with the leeks and the other ingredients, toss, divide into small cups and serve.

Nutrition: calories 280, fat 9.1, fiber 5.2, carbs 12.6, protein 5

Leeks Dip

Preparation time: 5 minutes
Cooking time: 0 minutes
Servings: 4

Ingredients:
- 1 tablespoon lemon juice
- ½ cup low-fat cream cheese
- 2 tablespoons olive oil
- Black pepper to the taste
- 4 leeks, chopped
- 1 tablespoon cilantro, chopped

Directions:
1. In a blender, combine the cream cheese with the leeks and the other ingredients, pulse well, divide into bowls and serve as a party dip.

Nutrition: calories 300, fat 12.2, fiber 7.6, carbs 14.7, protein 5.6

Bell Peppers Slaw

Preparation time: 5 minutes
Cooking time: 0 minutes
Servings: 4

Ingredients:
- ½ pound red bell pepper, cut into thin strips
- 3 green onions, chopped
- 1 tablespoon olive oil
- 2 teaspoons ginger, grated
- ½ teaspoon rosemary, dried
- 3 tablespoons balsamic vinegar

Directions:
1. In a salad bowl, mix the bell peppers with the onions and the other ingredients, toss, divide into small cups and serve.

Nutrition: calories 160, fat 6, fiber 3, carbs 10.9, protein 5.2

Avocado Spread

Preparation time: 4 minutes
Cooking time: 0 minutes
Servings: 4

Ingredients:
- 2 tablespoons dill, chopped
- 1 shallot, chopped
- 2 garlic cloves, minced
- 2 avocados, peeled, pitted and chopped
- 1 cup coconut cream
- 2 tablespoons olive oil
- 2 tablespoons lime juice
- Black pepper to the taste

Directions:
1. In a blender, combine the avocados with the shallots, garlic and the other ingredients, pulse well, divide into small bowls and serve as a snack.

Nutrition: calories 300, fat 22.3, fiber 6.4, carbs 42, protein 8.9

Corn Dip

Preparation time: 30 minutes
Cooking time: 0 minutes
Servings: 4

Ingredients:
- A pinch of cayenne pepper
- A pinch of black pepper
- 2 cups corn
- 1 cup coconut cream
- 2 tablespoons lemon juice
- 2 tablespoon avocado oil

Directions:
1. In a blender, combine the corn with the cream and the other ingredients, pulse well, divide into bowls and serve as a party dip.

Nutrition: calories 215, fat 16.2, fiber 3.8, carbs 18.4, protein 4

Beans Bars

Preparation time: 2 hours
Cooking time: 0 minutes
Servings: 12

Ingredients:
- 1 cup canned black beans, no-salt-added, drained
- 1 cup coconut flakes, unsweetened
- 1 cup low-fat butter
- ½ cup chia seeds
- ½ cup coconut cream

Directions:
1. In a blender, combine the beans with the coconut flakes and the other ingredients, pulse well, spread this into a square pan, press, keep in the fridge for 2 hours, slice into medium bars and serve.

Nutrition: calories 141, fat 7, fiber 5, carbs 16.2, protein 5

Pumpkin Seeds and Apple Chips Mix

Preparation time: 10 minutes
Cooking time: 2 hours
Servings: 4

Ingredients:
- Cooking spray
- 2 teaspoons nutmeg, ground
- 1 cup pumpkin seeds
- 2 apples, cored and thinly sliced

Directions:
1. Arrange the pumpkin seeds and the apple chips on a lined baking sheet, sprinkle the nutmeg all over, grease them with the spray, introduce in the oven and bake at 300 degrees F for 2 hours.
2. Divide into bowls and serve as a snack.

Nutrition: calories 80, fat 0, fiber 3, carbs 7, protein 4

Tomatoes and Yogurt Dip

Preparation time: 5 minutes
Cooking time: 0 minutes
Servings: 4

Ingredients:
- 2 cups fat-free Greek yogurt
- 1 tablespoon parsley, chopped
- ¼ cup canned tomatoes, no-salt-added, chopped
- 2 tablespoons chives, chopped
- Black pepper to the taste

Directions:
1. In a bowl, mix the yogurt with the parsley and the other ingredients, whisk well, divide into small bowls and serve as a party dip.

Nutrition: calories 78, fat 0, fiber 0.2, carbs 10.6, protein 8.2

Cayenne Beet Bowls

Preparation time: 10 minutes
Cooking time: 35 minutes
Servings: 2

Ingredients:
- 1 teaspoon cayenne pepper
- 2 beets, peeled and cubed
- 1 teaspoon rosemary, dried
- 1 tablespoon olive oil
- 2 teaspoons lime juice

Directions:
1. In a roasting pan, combine the beet bites with the cayenne and the other ingredients, toss, introduce in the oven, roast at 355 degrees F for 35 minutes, divide into small bowls and serve as a snack.

Nutrition: calories 170, fat 12.2, fiber 7, carbs 15.1, protein 6

Walnuts and Pecans Bowls

Preparation time: 10 minutes
Cooking time: 10 minutes
Servings: 4

Ingredients:
- 2 cup walnuts
- 1 cup pecans, chopped
- 1 teaspoon avocado oil
- ½ teaspoon sweet paprika

Directions:
1. Spread the grapes and pecans on a lined baking sheet, add the oil and the paprika, toss, and bake at 400 degrees F for 10 minutes.
2. Divide into bowls and serve as a snack.

Nutrition: calories 220, fat 12.4, fiber 3, carbs 12.9, protein 5.6

Parsley Salmon Muffins

Preparation time: 10 minutes
Cooking time: 25 minutes
Servings: 4

Ingredients:

- 1 cup low-fat mozzarella cheese, shredded
- 8 ounces smoked salmon, skinless, boneless, and chopped
- 1 cup almond flour
- 1 egg, whisked
- 1 teaspoon parsley, dried
- 1 garlic clove, minced
- Black pepper to the taste
- Cooking spray

Directions:

1. In a bowl, combine the salmon with the mozzarella and the other ingredients except the cooking spray and stir well.
2. Divide this mix into a muffin tray greased with the cooking spray, bake in the oven at 375 degrees F for 25 minutes and serve as a snack.

Nutrition: calories 273, fat 17, fiber 3.5, carbs 6.9, protein 21.8

Squash Balls

Preparation time: 10 minutes
Cooking time: 20 minutes
Servings: 8

Ingredients:
- A drizzle of olive oil
- 1 big butternut squash, peeled and minced
- 2 tablespoons cilantro, chopped
- 2 eggs, whisked
- ½ cup whole wheat flour
- Black pepper to the taste
- 2 shallots, chopped
- 2 garlic cloves, minced

Directions:
1. In a bowl, mix the squash with the cilantro and the other ingredients except the oil, stir well and shape medium balls out of this mix.
2. Arrange them on a lined baking sheet, grease them with the oil, bake at 400 degrees F for 10 minutes on each side, divide into bowls and serve.

Nutrition: calories 78, fat 3, fiber 0.9, carbs 10.8, protein 2.7

Cheesy Pearl Onion Bowls

Preparation time: 10 minutes
Cooking time: 30 minutes
Servings: 8

Ingredients:

- 20 white pearl onions, peeled
- 3 tablespoons parsley, chopped
- 1 tablespoon chives, chopped
- Black pepper to the taste
- 1 cup low-fat mozzarella, grated
- 1 tablespoon olive oil

Directions:

1. Spread the pearl onions on a lined baking sheet, add the oil, parsley, chives and the black pepper and toss.
2. Sprinkle the mozzarella on top, bake at 390 degrees F for 30 minutes, divide into bowls and serve cold as a snack.

Nutrition: calories 136, fat 2.7, fiber 6, carbs 25.9, protein 4.1

Broccoli Bars

Preparation time: 10 minutes
Cooking time: 25 minutes
Servings: 8

Ingredients:
- 1 pound broccoli florets, chopped
- ½ cup low-fat mozzarella cheese, shredded
- 2 eggs, whisked
- 1 teaspoon oregano, dried
- 1 teaspoon basil, dried
- Black pepper to the taste

Directions:
1. In a bowl, mix the broccoli with the cheese and the other ingredients, stir well, spread into a rectangle pan and press well on the bottom.
2. Introduce in the oven at 380 degrees F, bake for 25 minutes, cut into bars and serve cold.

Nutrition: calories 46, fat 1.3, fiber 1.8, carbs 4.2, protein 5

Pineapple and Tomato Salsa

Preparation time: 10 minutes
Cooking time: 40 minutes
Servings: 4

Ingredients:
- 20 ounces canned pineapple, drained and cubed
- 1 cup sun-dried tomatoes, cubed
- 1 tablespoon basil, chopped
- 1 tablespoon avocado oil
- 1 teaspoon lime juice
- 1 cup black olives, pitted and sliced
- Black pepper to the taste

Directions:
1. In a bowl, combine the pineapple cubes with the tomatoes and the other ingredients, toss, divide into smaller cups and serve as a snack.

Nutrition: calories 125, fat 4.3, fiber 3.8, carbs 23.6, protein 1.5

Turkey and Artichokes Mix

Preparation time: 5 minutes
Cooking time: 25 minutes
Servings: 4

Ingredients:
- 2 tablespoons olive oil
- 1 turkey breast, skinless, boneless and sliced
- A pinch of black pepper
- 1 tablespoon basil, chopped
- 3 garlic cloves, minced
- 14 ounces canned artichokes, no-salt-added, chopped
- 1 cup coconut cream
- ¾ cup low-fat mozzarella, shredded

Directions:
1. Heat up a pan with the oil over medium-high heat, add the meat, garlic and the black pepper, toss and cook for 5 minutes.
2. Add the rest of the ingredients except the cheese, toss and cook over medium heat for 15 minutes.
3. Sprinkle the cheese, cook everything for 5 minutes more, divide between plates and serve.

Nutrition: calories 300, fat 22.2, fiber 7.2, carbs 16.5, protein 13.6

Oregano Turkey Mix

Preparation time: 10 minutes
Cooking time: 30 minutes
Servings: 4

Ingredients:

- 2 tablespoons avocado oil
- 1 red onion, chopped
- 2 garlic cloves, minced
- A pinch of black pepper
- 1 tablespoon oregano, chopped
- 1 big turkey breast, skinless, boneless and cubed
- 1 and ½ cups low-sodium beef stock
- 1 tablespoon chives, chopped

Directions:

1. Heat up a pan with the oil over medium heat, add the onion, stir and sauté for 3 minutes.
2. Add the garlic and the meat, toss and cook for 3 minutes more.
3. Add the rest of the ingredients, toss, simmer everything over medium heat fro 25 minutes, divide between plates and serve.

Nutrition: calories 76, fat 2.1, fiber 1.7, carbs 6.4, protein 8.3

Orange Chicken

Preparation time: 10 minutes
Cooking time: 35 minutes
Servings: 4

Ingredients:
- 1 tablespoon avocado oil
- 1 pound chicken breast, skinless, boneless and halved
- 2 garlic cloves, minced
- 2 shallots, chopped
- ½ cup orange juice
- 1 tablespoon orange zest, grated
- 3 tablespoons balsamic vinegar
- 1 teaspoon rosemary, chopped

Directions:
1. Heat up a pan with the oil over medium-high heat, add the shallots and the garlic, toss and sauté for 2 minutes.
2. Add the meat, toss gently and cook for 3 minutes more.
3. Add the rest of the ingredients, toss, introduce the pan in the oven and bake at 340 degrees F for 30 minutes.
4. Divide between plates and serve.

Nutrition: calories 159, fat 3.4, fiber 0.5, carbs 5.4, protein 24.6

Garlic Turkey and Mushrooms

Preparation time: 10 minutes
Cooking time: 40 minutes
Servings: 4

Ingredients:
- 1 turkey breast, boneless, skinless and cubed
- ½ pound white mushrooms, halved
- 1/3 cup coconut aminos
- 2 garlic cloves, minced
- 2 tablespoons olive oil
- A pinch of black pepper
- 2 green onion, chopped
- 3 tablespoons garlic sauce
- 1 tablespoon rosemary, chopped

Directions:
1. Heat up a pan with the oil over medium heat, add the green onions, garlic sauce and the garlic and sauté for 5 minutes.
2. Add the meat and brown it for 5 minutes more.
3. Add the rest of the ingredients, introduce in the oven and bake at 390 degrees F for 30 minutes.
4. Divide the mix between plates and serve.

Nutrition: calories 154, fat 8.1, fiber 1.5, carbs 11.5, protein 9.8

Chicken and Olives Pan

Preparation time: 10 minutes
Cooking time: 25 minutes
Servings: 4

Ingredients:

- 1 pound chicken breasts, skinless, boneless and roughly cubed
- A pinch of black pepper
- 1 tablespoon avocado oil
- 1 red onion, chopped
- 1 cup coconut milk
- 1 tablespoon lemon juice
- 1 cup kalamata olives, pitted and sliced
- ¼ cup cilantro, chopped

Directions:

1. Heat up a pan with the oil over medium-high heat, add the onion and the meat and brown for 5 minutes.
2. Add the rest of the ingredients, toss, bring to a simmer and cook over medium heat for 20 minutes more.
3. Divide between plates and serve.

Nutrition: calories 409, fat 26.8, fiber 3.2, carbs 8.3, protein 34.9

Balsamic Turkey and Peach Mix

Preparation time: 10 minutes
Cooking time: 25 minutes
Servings: 4

Ingredients:
- 1 tablespoon avocado oil
- 1 turkey breast, skinless, boneless and sliced
- A pinch of black pepper
- 1 yellow onion, chopped
- 4 peaches, stones removed and cut into wedges
- ¼ cup balsamic vinegar
- 2 tablespoons chives, chopped

Directions:
1. Heat up a pan with the oil over medium-high heat, add the meat and the onion, toss and brown for 5 minutes.
2. Add the rest of the ingredients except the chives, toss gently and bake at 390 degrees F for 20 minutes.
3. Divide everything between plates and serve with the chives sprinkled on top.

Nutrition: calories 123, fat 1.6, fiber 3.3, carbs 18.8, protein 9.1

Coconut Chicken and Spinach

Preparation time: 10 minutes
Cooking time: 25 minutes
Servings: 4

Ingredients:
- 1 tablespoon avocado oil
- 1 pound chicken breast, skinless, boneless and cubed
- ½ teaspoon basil, dried
- A pinch of black pepper
- ¼ cup low-sodium veggie stock
- 2 cups baby spinach
- 2 shallots, chopped
- 2 garlic cloves, minced
- ½ teaspoon sweet paprika
- 2/3 cup coconut cream
- 2 tablespoons cilantro, chopped

Directions:
1. Heat up a pan with the oil over medium-high heat, add the meat, basil, black pepper and brown for 5 minutes.
2. Add the shallots and the garlic and cook for another 5 minutes.
3. Add the rest of the ingredients, toss, bring to a simmer and cook over medium heat fro 15 minutes more.
4. Divide between plates and serve hot.

Nutrition: calories 237, fat 12.9, fiber 1.6, carbs 4.7, protein 25.8

Chicken and Asparagus Mix

Preparation time: 10 minutes
Cooking time: 25 minutes
Servings: 4

Ingredients:

- 2 chicken breasts, skinless, boneless and cubed
- 2 tablespoons avocado oil
- 2 spring onions, chopped
- 1 bunch asparagus, trimmed and halved
- ½ teaspoon sweet paprika
- A pinch of black pepper
- 14 ounces canned tomatoes, no-salt-added, drained and chopped

Directions:

1. Heat up a pan with the oil over medium-high heat, add the meat and the spring onions, stir and cook for 5 minutes.
2. Add the asparagus and the other ingredients, toss, cover the pan and cook over medium heat for 20 minutes.
3. Divide everything between plates and serve.

Nutrition: calories 171, fat 6.4, fiber 2,6, carbs 6.4, protein 22.2

Turkey and Creamy Broccoli

Preparation time: 10 minutes
Cooking time: 25 minutes
Servings: 4

Ingredients:
- 1 tablespoon olive oil
- 1 big turkey breast, skinless, boneless and cubed
- 2 cups broccoli florets
- 2 shallots, chopped
- 2 garlic cloves, minced
- 1 tablespoon basil, chopped
- 1 tablespoon cilantro, chopped
- ½ cup coconut cream

Directions:
1. Heat up a pan with the oil over medium-high heat, add the meat, shallots and the garlic, toss and brown for 5 minutes.
2. Add the broccoli and the other ingredients, toss everything, cook for 20 minutes over medium heat, divide between plates and serve.

Nutrition: calories 165, fat 11.5, fiber 2.1, carbs 7.9, protein 9.6

Chicken and Dill Green Beans Mix

Preparation time: 10 minutes
Cooking time: 25 minutes
Servings: 4

Ingredients:

- 2 tablespoons olive oil
- 10 ounces green beans, trimmed and halved
- 1 yellow onion, chopped
- 1 tablespoon dill, chopped
- 2 chicken breasts, skinless, boneless and halved
- 2 cups tomato sauce, no-salt-added
- ½ teaspoon red pepper flakes, crushed

Directions:

1. Heat up a pan with the oil over medium-high heat, add the onion and the meat and brown it for 2 minutes on each side.
2. Add the green beans and the other ingredients, toss, introduce in the oven and bake at 380 degrees F fro 20 minutes.
3. Divide between plates and serve right away.

Nutrition: calories 391, fat 17.8, fiber 5, carbs 14.8, protein 43.9

Chicken and Chili Zucchini

Preparation time: 5 minutes
Cooking time: 25 minutes
Servings: 4

Ingredients:

- 1 pound chicken breasts, skinless, boneless and cubed
- 1 cup low-sodium chicken stock
- 2 zucchinis, roughly cubed
- 1 tablespoon olive oil
- 1 cup canned tomatoes, no-salt-added, chopped
- 1 yellow onion, chopped
- 1 teaspoon chili powder
- 1 tablespoon cilantro, chopped

Directions:

1. Heat up a pan with the oil over medium-high heat, add the meat and the onion, toss and brown for 5 minutes.
2. Add the zucchinis and the rest of the ingredients, toss gently, reduce the heat to medium and cook for 20 minutes.
3. Divide everything between plates and serve.

Nutrition: calories 284, fat 12.3, fiber 2.4, carbs 8, protein 35

Avocado and Chicken Mix

Preparation time: 10 minutes
Cooking time: 20 minutes
Servings: 4

Ingredients:
- 2 chicken breasts, skinless, boneless and halved
- Juice of ½ lemon
- 2 tablespoons olive oil
- 2 garlic cloves, minced
- ½ cup low-sodium veggie stock
- 1 avocado, peeled, pitted and cut into wedges
- A pinch of black pepper

Directions:
1. Heat up a pan with the oil over medium heat, add the garlic and the meat and brown for 2 minutes on each side.
2. Add the lemon juice and the other ingredients, bring to a simmer and cook over medium heat fro 15 minutes.
3. Divide the whole mix between plates and serve.

Nutrition: calories 436, fat 27.3, fiber 3.6, carbs 5.6, protein 41.8

Turkey and Bok Choy

Preparation time: 10 minutes
Cooking time: 20 minutes
Servings: 4

Ingredients:

- 1 turkey breast, boneless, skinless and roughly cubed
- 2 scallions, chopped
- 1 pound bok choy, torn
- 2 tablespoons olive oil
- ½ teaspoon ginger, grated
- A pinch of black pepper
- ½ cup low-sodium veggie stock

Directions:

1. Heat up a pot with the oil over medium-high heat, add the scallions and the ginger and sauté for 2 minutes.
2. Add the meat and brown for 5 minutes more.
3. Add the rest of the ingredients, toss, simmer for 13 minutes more, divide between plates and serve.

Nutrition: calories 125, fat 8, fiber 1.7, carbs 5.5, protein 9.3

Chicken with Red Onion Mix

Preparation time: 10 minutes
Cooking time: 25 minutes
Servings: 4

Ingredients:
- 2 chicken breasts, skinless, boneless and roughly cubed
- 3 red onions, sliced
- 2 tablespoons olive oil
- 1 cup low-sodium veggie stock
- A pinch of black pepper
- 1 tablespoon cilantro, chopped
- 1 tablespoon chives, chopped

Directions:
1. Heat up a pan with the oil over medium heat, add the onions and a pinch of black pepper, and sauté for 10 minutes stirring often.
2. Add the chicken and cook for 3 minutes more.
3. Add the rest of the ingredients, bring to a simmer and cook over medium heat for 12 minutes more.
4. Divide the chicken and onions mix between plates and serve.

Nutrition: calories 364, fat 17.5, fiber 2.1, carbs 8.8, protein 41.7

Hot Turkey and Rice

Preparation time: 10 minutes
Cooking time: 42 minutes
Servings: 4

Ingredients:
- 1 turkey breast, skinless, boneless and cubed
- 1 cup white rice
- 2 cups low-sodium veggie stock
- 1 teaspoon hot paprika
- 2 small Serrano peppers, chopped
- 2 garlic cloves, minced
- 2 tablespoons olive oil
- ½ red bell pepper chopped
- A pinch of black pepper

Directions:
1. Heat up a pan with the oil over medium heat, add the Serrano peppers and garlic and sauté for 2 minutes.
2. Add the meat and brown it for 5 minutes.
3. Add the rice and the other ingredients, bring to a simmer and cook over medium heat for 35 minutes.
4. Stir, divide between plates and serve.

Nutrition: calories 271, fat 7.7, fiber 1.7, carbs 42, protein 7.8

Lemony Leek and Chicken

Preparation time: 10 minutes
Cooking time: 40 minutes
Servings: 4

Ingredients:
- 1 pound chicken breast, skinless, boneless and cubed
- A pinch of black pepper
- 2 tablespoons avocado oil
- 1 tablespoon tomato sauce, no-salt-added
- 1 cup low-sodium veggie stock
- 4 leek, roughly chopped
- ½ cup lemon juice

Directions:
1. Heat up a pan with the oil over medium heat, add the leeks, toss and sauté for 10 minutes.
2. Add the chicken and the other ingredients, toss, cook over medium heat for 20 minutes more, divide between plates and serve.

Nutrition: calories 199, fat 13.3, fiber 5, carbs 7.6, protein 17.4

Turkey with Savoy Cabbage Mix

Preparation time: 10 minutes
Cooking time: 35 minutes
Servings: 4

Ingredients:
- 1 big turkey breast, skinless, boneless and cubed
- 1 cup low-sodium chicken stock
- 1 tablespoon coconut oil, melted
- 1 Savoy cabbage, shredded
- 1 teaspoon chili powder
- 1 teaspoon sweet paprika
- 1 garlic clove, minced
- 1 yellow onion, chopped
- A pinch of salt and black pepper

Directions:
1. Heat up a pan with the oil over medium heat, add the meat and brown for 5 minutes.
2. Add the garlic and the onion, toss and sauté for 5 minutes more.
3. Add the cabbage and the other ingredients, toss, bring to a simmer and cook over medium heat for 25 minutes.
4. Divide everything between plates and serve.

Nutrition: calories 299, fat 14.5, fiber 5, carbs 8.8, protein 12.6

Chicken with Paprika Scallions

Preparation time: 10 minutes
Cooking time: 30 minutes
Servings: 4

Ingredients:
- 1 pound chicken breast, skinless, boneless and sliced
- 4 scallions, chopped
- 1 tablespoon olive oil
- 1 tablespoon sweet paprika
- 1 cup low-sodium chicken stock
- 1 tablespoon ginger, grated
- 1 teaspoon oregano, dried
- 1 teaspoon cumin, ground
- 1 teaspoon allspice, ground
- ½ cup cilantro, chopped
- A pinch of black pepper

Directions:
1. Heat up a pan with the oil over medium heat, add the scallions and the meat and brown for 5 minutes.
2. Add the rest of the ingredients, toss, introduce in the oven and bake at 390 degrees F for 25 minutes.
3. Divide the chicken and scallions mix between plates and serve.

Nutrition: calories 295, fat 12.5, fiber 6.9, carbs 22.4, protein 15.6

Chicken and Mustard Sauce

Preparation time: 10 minutes
Cooking time: 35 minutes
Servings: 4

Ingredients:

- 1 pound chicken thighs, boneless and skinless
- 1 tablespoon avocado oil
- 2 tablespoons mustard
- 1 shallot, chopped
- 1 cup low-sodium chicken stock
- A pinch of salt and black pepper
- 3 garlic cloves, minced
- ½ teaspoon basil, dried

Directions:

1. Heat up a pan with the oil over medium heat, add the shallot, garlic and the chicken and brown everything for 5 minutes.
2. Add the mustard and the rest of the ingredients, toss gently, bring to a simmer and cook over medium heat for 30 minutes.
3. Divide everything between plates and serve hot.

Nutrition: calories 299, fat 15.5, fiber 6.6, carbs 30.3, protein 12.5

Chicken and Celery Mix

Preparation time: 10 minutes
Cooking time: 35 minutes
Servings: 4

Ingredients:
- A pinch of black pepper
- 2 pounds chicken breast, skinless, boneless and cubed
- 2 tablespoons olive oil
- 1 cup celery, chopped
- 3 garlic cloves, minced
- 1 poblano pepper, chopped
- 1 cup low-sodium veggie stock
- 1 teaspoon chili powder
- 2 tablespoons chives, chopped

Directions:
1. Heat up a pan with the oil over medium heat, add the garlic, celery and poblano pepper, toss and cook for 5 minutes.
2. Add the meat, toss and cook for another 5 minutes.
3. Add the rest of the ingredients except the chives, bring to a simmer and cook over medium heat for 25 minutes more.
4. Divide the whole mix between plates and serve with the chives sprinkled on top.

Nutrition: calories 305, fat 18, fiber 13.4, carbs 22.5, protein 6

Lime Turkey with Baby Potatoes

Preparation time: 10 minutes
Cooking time: 40 minutes
Servings: 4

Ingredients:
- 1 turkey breast, skinless, boneless and sliced
- 2 tablespoons olive oil
- 1 pound baby potatoes, peeled and halved
- 1 tablespoon sweet paprika
- 1 yellow onion, chopped
- 1 teaspoon chili powder
- 1 teaspoon rosemary, dried
- 2 cups low-sodium chicken stock
- A pinch of black pepper
- Zest of 1 lime, grated
- 1 tablespoon lime juice
- 1 tablespoon cilantro, chopped

Directions:

1. Heat up a pan with the oil over medium heat, add the onion, chili powder and the rosemary, toss and sauté for 5 minutes.
2. Add the meat, and brown for 5 minutes more.
3. Add the potatoes and the rest of the ingredients except the cilantro, toss gently, bring to a simmer and cook over medium heat for 30 minutes.
4. Divide the mix between plates and serve with the cilantro sprinkled on top.

Nutrition: calories 345, fat 22.2, fiber 12.3, carbs 34.5, protein 16.4

Chicken with Mustard Greens

Preparation time: 10 minutes
Cooking time: 25 minutes
Servings: 4

Ingredients:
- 2 chicken breasts, skinless, boneless and cubed
- 3 cups mustard greens
- 1 cup canned tomatoes, no-salt-added, chopped
- 1 red onion, chopped
- 2 tablespoons avocado oil
- 1 teaspoon oregano, dried
- 2 garlic cloves, minced
- 1 tablespoon chives, chopped
- 1 tablespoon balsamic vinegar
- A pinch of black pepper

Directions:
1. Heat up a pan with the oil over medium-high heat, add the onion and the garlic and sauté for 5 minutes.
2. Add the meat and brown it for 5 minutes more.
3. Add the greens, tomatoes and the other ingredients, toss, cook for 20 minutes over medium heat, divide between plates and serve.

Nutrition: calories 290, fat 12.3, fiber 6.7, carbs 22.30, protein 14.3

Baked Chicken and Apples

Preparation time: 10 minutes
Cooking time: 50 minutes
Servings: 4

Ingredients:

- 2 pounds chicken thighs, boneless and skinless
- 2 tablespoons olive oil
- 2 red onions, sliced
- A pinch of black pepper
- 1 teaspoon thyme, dried
- 1 teaspoon basil, dried
- 1 cup green apples, cored and roughly cubed
- 2 garlic cloves, minced
- 2 cups low-sodium chicken stock
- 1 tablespoon lemon juice
- 1 cup tomatoes, cubed
- 1 tablespoon cilantro, chopped

Directions:

1. Heat up a pan with the oil over medium-high heat, add the onions and garlic, and sauté for 5 minutes.
2. Add the chicken and brown for another 5 minutes.
3. Add the thyme, basil and the other ingredients, toss gently, introduce in the oven and bake at 390 degrees F for 40 minutes.
4. Divide the chicken and apples mix between plates and serve.

Nutrition: calories 290, fat 12.3, fiber 4, carbs 15.7, protein 10

Chipotle Chicken

Preparation time: 10 minutes
Cooking time: 1 hour
Servings: 6

Ingredients:
- 2 pounds chicken thighs, boneless and skinless
- 1 yellow onion, chopped
- 2 tablespoons olive oil
- 3 garlic cloves, minced
- 1 tablespoon coriander seeds, ground
- 1 teaspoon cumin, ground
- 1 cup low-sodium chicken stock
- 4 tablespoons chipotle chili paste
- A pinch of black pepper
- 1 tablespoon coriander, chopped

Directions:

1. Heat up a pan with the oil over medium heat, add the onion and the garlic and sauté for 5 minutes.
2. Add the meat and brown for 5 minutes more.
3. Add the rest of the ingredients, toss, introduce everything in the oven and bake at 390 degrees F for 50 minutes.
4. Divide the whole mix between plates and serve.

Nutrition: calories 280, fat 12.1, fiber 6.3, carbs 15.7, protein 12

Herbed Turkey

Preparation time: 10 minutes
Cooking time: 35 minutes
Servings: 4

Ingredients:
- 1 big turkey breast, boneless, skinless and sliced
- 1 tablespoon chives, chopped
- 1 tablespoon oregano, chopped
- 1 tablespoon basil, chopped
- 1 tablespoon coriander, chopped
- 2 shallots, chopped
- 2 tablespoons olive oil
- 1 cup low-sodium chicken stock
- 1 cup tomatoes, cubed
- Salt and black pepper to the taste

Directions:
1. Heat up a pan with the oil over medium heat, add the shallots and the meat and brown for 5 minutes.
2. Add the chives and the other ingredients, toss, bring to a simmer and cook over medium heat for 30 minutes.
3. Divide the mix between plates and serve.

Nutrition: calories 290, fat 11.9, fiber 5.5, carbs 16.2, protein 9

Chicken and Ginger Sauce

Preparation time: 10 minutes
Cooking time: 35 minutes
Servings: 4

Ingredients:
- 1 pound chicken breast, skinless, boneless and cubed
- 1 tablespoon ginger, grated
- 1 tablespoon olive oil
- 2 shallots, chopped
- 1 tablespoon balsamic vinegar
- A pinch of black pepper
- ¾ cup low-sodium chicken stock
- 1 tablespoon basil, chopped

Directions:
1. Heat up a pan with the oil over medium heat, add the shallots and the ginger, stir and sauté for 5 minutes.
2. Add the rest of the ingredients except the chicken, toss, bring to a simmer and cook for 5 minutes more.
3. Add the chicken, toss, simmer the whole mix for 25 minutes, divide between plates and serve.

Nutrition: calories 294, fat 15.5, fiber 3, carbs 15.4, protein 13.1

Chicken and Corn

Preparation time: 10 minutes
Cooking time: 35 minutes
Servings: 4

Ingredients:

- 2 pounds chicken breast, skinless, boneless and halved
- 2 cups corn
- 2 tablespoons avocado oil
- A pinch of black pepper
- 1 teaspoon smoked paprika
- 1 bunch green onions, chopped
- 1 cup low-sodium chicken stock

Directions:

1. Heat up a pan with the oil over medium-high heat, add the green onions, stir and sauté them for 5 minutes.
2. Add the chicken and brown it for 5 minutes more.
3. Add the corn and the other ingredients, toss, introduce the pan in the oven and cook at 390 degrees F for 25 minutes.
4. Divide the mix between plates and serve.

Nutrition: calories 270, fat 12.4, fiber 5.2, carbs 12, protein 9

Curry Turkey and Quinoa

Preparation time: 10 minutes
Cooking time: 40 minutes
Servings: 4

Ingredients:
- 1 pound turkey breast, skinless, boneless and cubed
- 1 tablespoon olive oil
- 1 cup quinoa
- 2 cups low-sodium chicken stock
- 1 tablespoon lime juice
- 1 tablespoon parsley, chopped
- A pinch of black pepper
- 1 tablespoon red curry paste

Directions:
1. Heat up a pan with the oil over medium-high heat, add the meat and brown it for 5 minutes.
2. Add the quinoa and the rest of the ingredients, toss, bring to a simmer and cook over medium heat for 35 minutes.
3. Divide everything between plates and serve.

Nutrition: calories 310, fat 8.5, fiber 11, carbs 30.4, protein 16.3

Turkey and Cumin Parsnips

Preparation time: 10 minutes
Cooking time: 40 minutes
Servings: 4

Ingredients:

- 1 pound turkey breast, skinless, boneless and cubed
- 2 parsnips, peeled and cubed
- 2 teaspoons cumin, ground
- 1 tablespoon parsley, chopped
- 2 tablespoons avocado oil
- 2 shallots, chopped
- 1 cup low-sodium chicken stock
- 4 garlic cloves, minced
- A pinch of black pepper

Directions:

1. Heat up a pan with the oil over medium heat, add the shallots and the garlic and sauté for 5 minutes.
2. Add the turkey, toss and cook for 5 minutes more.
3. Add the parsnips and the other ingredients, toss, simmer over medium heat for 30 minutes more, divide between plates and serve.

Nutrition: calories 284, fat 18.2, fiber 4, carbs 16.7, protein 12.3

Turkey and Cilantro Chickpeas

Preparation time: 10 minutes
Cooking time: 40 minutes
Servings: 4

Ingredients:
- 1 cup canned chickpeas, no-salt-added, drained
- 1 cup low-sodium chicken stock
- 1 pound turkey breast, skinless, boneless and cubed
- A pinch of black pepper
- 1 teaspoon oregano, dried
- 1 teaspoon nutmeg, ground
- 2 tablespoons olive oil
- 1 yellow onion, chopped
- 1 green bell pepper, chopped
- 1 cup cilantro, chopped

Directions:
1. Heat up a pan with the oil over medium heat, add the onion, bell pepper and the meat and cook for 10 minutes stirring often.
2. Add the rest of the ingredients, toss, bring to a simmer and cook over medium heat for 30 minutes.
3. Divide the mix between plates and serve.

Nutrition: calories 304, fat 11.2, fiber 4.5, carbs 22.2, protein 17

Turkey and Curry Lentils

Preparation time: 10 minutes
Cooking time: 40 minutes
Servings: 4

Ingredients:
- 2 pounds turkey breast, skinless, boneless and cubed
- 1 cup canned lentils, no-salt-added, drained and rinsed
- 1 tablespoon green curry paste
- 1 teaspoon garam masala
- 2 tablespoons olive oil
- 1 yellow onion, chopped
- 1 garlic clove, minced
- A pinch of black pepper
- 1 tablespoon cilantro, chopped

Directions:
1. Heat up a pan with the oil over medium heat, add the onion, garlic and the meat and brown for 5 minutes stirring often.
2. Add the lentils and the other ingredients, bring to a simmer and cook over medium heat for 35 minutes.
3. Divide the mix between plates and serve.

Nutrition: calories 489, fat 12.1, fiber 16.4, carbs 42.4, protein 51.5

Turkey with Beans and Olives

Preparation time: 10 minutes
Cooking time: 35 minutes
Servings: 4

Ingredients:
- 1 cup black beans, no-salt-added and drained
- 1 cup green olives, pitted and halved
- 1 pound turkey breast, skinless, boneless and sliced
- 1 tablespoon cilantro, chopped
- 1 cup tomato sauce, no-salt-added
- 1 tablespoon olive oil

Directions:
1. Grease a baking dish with the oil, arrange the turkey slices inside, add the other ingredients as well, introduce in the oven and bake at 380 degrees F for 35 minutes.
2. Divide between plates and serve.

Nutrition: calories 331, fat 6.4, fiber 9, carbs 38.5, protein 30.7

Chicken and Tomato Quinoa

Preparation time: 10 minutes
Cooking time: 35 minutes
Servings: 8

Ingredients:
- 1 tablespoon olive oil
- 2 pounds chicken breasts, skinless, boneless and halved
- 1 teaspoon rosemary, ground
- A pinch of salt and black pepper
- 2 shallots, chopped
- 1 tablespoon olive oil
- 3 tablespoons low-sodium tomato sauce
- 2 cups quinoa, already cooked

Directions:
1. Heat up a pan with the oil over medium-high heat, add the meat and shallots and brown for 2 minutes on each side.
2. Add the rosemary and the other ingredients, toss, introduce in the oven and cook at 370 degrees F for 30 minutes.
3. Divide the mix between plates and serve.

Nutrition: calories 406, fat 14.5, fiber 3.1, carbs 28.1, protein 39

Allspice Chicken Wings

Preparation time: 10 minutes
Cooking time: 20 minutes
Servings: 4

Ingredients:
- 2 pounds chicken wings
- 2 teaspoons allspice, ground
- 2 tablespoons avocado oil
- 5 garlic cloves, minced
- Black pepper to the taste
- 2 tablespoons chives, chopped

Directions:
1. In a bowl, combine the chicken wings with the allspice and the other ingredients and toss well.
2. Arrange the chicken wings in a roasting pan and bake at 400 degrees F for 20 minutes.
3. Divide the chicken wings between plates and serve.

Nutrition: calories 449, fat 17.8, fiber 0.6, carbs 2.4, protein 66.1

Chicken and Snow Peas

Preparation time: 10 minutes
Cooking time: 30 minutes
Servings: 4

Ingredients:
- 2 pounds chicken breasts, skinless, boneless and cubed
- 2 cups snow peas
- 2 tablespoons olive oil
- 1 red onion, chopped
- 1 cup canned tomato sauce, no-salt-added
- 2 tablespoons parsley, chopped
- A pinch of black pepper

Directions:
1. Heat up a pan with the oil over medium heat, add the onion and the meat and brown for 5 minutes.
2. Add the peas and the rest of the ingredients, bring to a simmer and cook over medium heat for 25 minutes.
3. Divide the mix between plates and serve.

Nutrition: calories 551, fat 24.2, fiber 3.8, carbs 11.7, protein 69.4

Shrimp and Pineapple mix

Preparation time: 10 minutes
Cooking time: 10 minutes
Servings: 4

Ingredients:
- 1 tablespoon olive oil
- 1 pound shrimp, peeled and deveined
- 1 cup pineapple, peeled and cubed
- Juice of 1 lemon
- A bunch of parsley, chopped

Directions:
1. Heat up a pan with the oil over medium heat, add the shrimp and cook for 3 minutes on each side.
2. Add the rest of the ingredients, cook everything for 4 minutes more, divide into bowls and serve.

Nutrition: calories 254, fat 13.3, fiber 6, carbs 14.9, protein 11

Salmon and Green Olives

Preparation time: 10 minutes
Cooking time: 20 minutes
Servings: 4

Ingredients:
- 1 yellow onion, chopped
- 1 cup green olives, pitted and halved
- 1 teaspoon chili powder
- Black pepper to the taste
- 2 tablespoons olive oil
- ¼ cup low-sodium veggie stock
- 4 salmon fillets, skinless and boneless
- 2 tablespoons chives, chopped

Directions:
1. Heat up a pan with the oil over medium-high heat, add the onion and sauté for 3 minutes.
2. Add the salmon and cook for 5 minutes on each side. Add the rest of the ingredients, cook the mix for 5 minutes more, divide between plates and serve.

Nutrition: calories 221, fat 12.1, fiber 5.4, carbs 8.5, protein 11.2

Salmon and Fennel

Preparation time: 5 minutes
Cooking time: 15 minutes
Servings: 4

Ingredients:
- 4 medium salmon fillets, skinless and boneless
- 1 fennel bulb, chopped
- ½ cup low-sodium veggie stock
- 2 tablespoons olive oil
- Black pepper to the taste
- ¼ cup low-sodium veggie stock
- 1 tablespoon lemon juice
- 1 tablespoon cilantro, chopped

Directions:
1. Heat up a pan with the oil over medium heat, add the fennel and cook for 3 minutes.
2. Add the fish and brown it for 4 minutes on each side.
3. Add the rest of the ingredients, cook everything for 4 minutes more, divide between plates and serve.

Nutrition: calories 252, fat 9.3, fiber 4.2, carbs 12.3, protein 9

Cod and Asparagus

Preparation time: 10 minutes
Cooking time: 14 minutes
Servings: 4

Ingredients:

- 1 tablespoon olive oil
- 1 red onion, chopped
- 1 pound cod fillets, boneless
- 1 bunch asparagus, trimmed
- Black pepper to the taste
- 1 cup coconut cream
- 1 tablespoon chives, chopped

Directions:

1. Heat up a pan with the oil over medium heat, add the onion and the cod and cook it for 3 minutes on each side.
2. Add the rest of the ingredients, cook everything for 8 minutes more, divide between plates and serve.

Nutrition: calories 254, fat 12.1, fiber 5.4, carbs 4.2, protein 13.5

Spiced Shrimp

Preparation time: 5 minutes
Cooking time: 8 minutes
Servings: 4

Ingredients:
- 1 teaspoon garlic powder
- 1 teaspoon smoked paprika
- 1 teaspoon cumin, ground
- 1 teaspoon allspice, ground
- 2 tablespoons olive oil
- 2 pounds shrimp, peeled and deveined
- 1 tablespoon chives, chopped

Directions:
1. Heat up a pan with the oil over medium heat, add the shrimp, garlic powder and the other ingredients, cook for 4 minutes on each side, divide into bowls and serve.

Nutrition: calories 212, fat 9.6, fiber 5.3, carbs 12.7, protein 15.4

Sea Bass and Tomatoes

Preparation time: 10 minutes
Cooking time: 30 minutes
Servings: 4

Ingredients:

- 2 tablespoons olive oil
- 2 pounds sea bass fillets, skinless and boneless
- Black pepper to the taste
- 2 cups cherry tomatoes, halved
- 1 tablespoon chives, chopped
- 1 tablespoon lemon zest, grated
- ¼ cup lemon juice

Directions:

1. Grease a roasting pan with the oil and arrange the fish inside.
2. Add the tomatoes and the other ingredients, introduce the pan in the oven and bake at 380 degrees F for 30 minutes.
3. Divide everything between plates and serve.

Nutrition: calories 272, fat 6.9, fiber 6.2, carbs 18.4, protein 9

Shrimp and Beans

Preparation time: 10 minutes
Cooking time: 12 minutes
Servings: 4

Ingredients:
- 1 pound shrimp, deveined and peeled
- 1 tablespoon olive oil
- Juice of 1 lime
- 1 cup canned black beans, no-salt-added, drained
- 1 shallot, chopped
- 1 tablespoon oregano, chopped
- 2 garlic cloves, chopped
- Black pepper to the taste

Directions:
1. Heat up a pan with the oil over medium-high heat, add the shallot and the garlic, stir and cook for 3 minutes.
2. Add the shrimp and cook for 2 minutes on each side.
3. Add the beans and the other ingredients, cook everything over medium heat for 5 minutes more, divide into bowls and serve.

Nutrition: calories 253, fat 11.6, fiber 6, carbs 14.5, protein 13.5

Shrimp and Horseradish Mix

Preparation time: 5 minutes
Cooking time: 8 minutes
Servings: 4

Ingredients:
- 1 pound shrimp, peeled and deveined
- 2 shallots, chopped
- 1 tablespoon olive oil
- 1 tablespoon chives, chopped
- 2 teaspoons prepared horseradish
- ¼ cup coconut cream
- Black pepper to the taste

Directions:
4 Heat up a pan with the oil over medium heat, add the shallots and the horseradish, stir and sauté for 2 minutes.
5 Add the shrimp and the other ingredients, toss, cook for 6 minutes more, divide between plates and serve.

Nutrition: calories 233, fat 6, fiber 5, carbs 11.9, protein 5.4

Shrimp and Tarragon Salad

Preparation time: 4 minutes
Cooking time: 0 minutes
Servings: 4

Ingredients:
- 1 pound shrimp, cooked, peeled and deveined
- 1 tablespoon tarragon, chopped
- 1 tablespoon capers, drained
- 2 tablespoons olive oil
- Black pepper to the taste
- 2 cups baby spinach
- 1 tablespoon balsamic vinegar
- 1 small red onion, sliced
- 2 tablespoons lemon juice

Directions:
4 In a bowl, combine the shrimp with the tarragon and the other ingredients, toss and serve.

Nutrition: calories 258, fat 12.4, fiber 6, carbs 6.7, protein 13.3

Parmesan Cod Mix

Preparation time: 10 minutes
Cooking time: 20 minutes
Servings: 4

Ingredients:
- 4 cod fillets, boneless
- ½ cup low-fat parmesan cheese, shredded
- 3 garlic cloves, minced
- 1 tablespoon olive oil
- 1 tablespoon lemon juice
- ½ cup green onion, chopped

Directions:
1. Heat up a pan with the oil over medium heat, add the garlic and the green onions, toss and sauté for 5 minutes.
2. Add the fish and cook it for 4 minutes on each side.
3. Add the lemon juice, sprinkle the parmesan on top, cook everything for 2 minutes more, divide between plates and serve.

Nutrition: calories 275, fat 22.1, fiber 5, carbs 18.2, protein 12

Tilapia and Red Onion Mix

Preparation time: 10 minutes
Cooking time: 15 minutes
Servings: 4

Ingredients:
- 4 tilapia fillets, boneless
- 2 tablespoons olive oil
- 1 tablespoon lemon juice
- 2 teaspoons lemon zest, grated
- 2 red onions, roughly chopped
- 3 tablespoons chives, chopped

Directions:
1. Heat up a pan with the oil over medium heat, add the onions, lemon zest and lemon juice, toss and sauté for 5 minutes.
2. Add the fish and the chives, cook for 5 minutes on each side, divide between plates and serve.

Nutrition: calories 254, fat 18.2, fiber 5.4, carbs 11.7, protein 4.5

Trout Salad

Preparation time: 6 minutes
Cooking time: 0 minutes
Servings: 4

Ingredients:

- 4 ounces smoked trout, skinless, boneless and cubed
- 1 tablespoon lime juice
- 1/3 cup non-fat yogurt
- 2 avocados, peeled, pitted and cubed
- 3 tablespoons chives, chopped
- Black pepper to the taste
- 1 tablespoon olive oil

Directions:

1. In a bowl, combine the trout with the avocados and the other ingredients, toss, and serve.

Nutrition: calories 244, fat 9.45, fiber 5.6, carbs 8.5, protein 15

Balsamic Trout

Preparation time: 5 minutes
Cooking time: 15 minutes
Servings: 4

Ingredients:
- 3 tablespoons balsamic vinegar
- 2 tablespoons olive oil
- 4 trout fillets, boneless
- 3 tablespoons parsley, finely chopped
- 2 garlic cloves, minced

Directions:
1. Heat up a pan with the oil over medium heat, add the trout and cook for 6 minutes on each side.
2. Add the rest of the ingredients, cook for 3 minutes more, divide between plates and serve with a side salad.

Nutrition: calories 314, fat 14.3, fiber 8.2, carbs 14.8, protein 11.2

Parsley Salmon

Preparation time: 5 minutes
Cooking time: 12 minutes
Servings: 4

Ingredients:

- 2 spring onions, chopped
- 2 teaspoons lime juice
- 1 tablespoon chives, minced
- 1 tablespoon olive oil
- 4 salmon fillets, boneless
- Black pepper to the taste
- 2 tablespoons parsley, chopped

Directions:

1. Heat up a pan with the oil over medium heat, add the spring onions, stir and sauté for 2 minutes.
2. Add the salmon and the other ingredients, cook for 5 minutes on each side, divide between plates and serve.

Nutrition: calories 290, fat 14.4, fiber 5.6, carbs 15.6, protein 9.5

Trout and Veggie Salad

Preparation time: 5 minutes
Cooking time: 0 minutes
Servings: 4

Ingredients:

- 2 tablespoons olive oil
- ½ cup kalamata olives, pitted and minced
- Black pepper to the taste
- 1 pound smoked trout, boneless, skinless and cubed
- ½ teaspoon lemon zest, grated
- 1 tablespoon lemon juice
- 1 cup cherry tomatoes, halved
- ½ red onion, sliced
- 2 cups baby arugula

Directions:

1. In a bowl, combine smoked trout with the olives, black pepper and the other ingredients, toss and serve.

Nutrition: calories 282, fat 13.4, fiber 5.3, carbs 11.6, protein 5.6

Saffron Salmon

Preparation time: 10 minutes
Cooking time: 12 minutes
Servings: 4

Ingredients:
- Black pepper to the taste
- ½ teaspoon sweet paprika
- 4 salmon fillets, boneless
- 3 tablespoons olive oil
- 1 yellow onion, chopped
- 2 garlic cloves, minced
- ¼ teaspoon saffron powder

Directions:
1. Heat up a pan with the oil over medium-high heat, add the onion and the garlic, toss and sauté for 2 minutes.
2. Add the salmon and the other ingredients, cook for 5 minutes on each side, divide between plates and serve.

Nutrition: calories 339, fat 21.6, fiber 0.7, carbs 3.2, protein 35

Shrimp and Watermelon Salad

Preparation time: 10 minutes
Cooking time: 0 minutes
Servings: 4

Ingredients:
- ¼ cup basil, chopped
- 2 cups watermelon, peeled and cubed
- 2 tablespoons balsamic vinegar
- 2 tablespoons olive oil
- 1 pound shrimp, peeled, deveined and cooked
- Black pepper to the taste
- 1 tablespoon parsley, chopped

Directions:
1. In a bowl, combine the shrimp with the watermelon and the other ingredients, toss and serve.

Nutrition: calories 220, fat 9, fiber 0.4, carbs 7.6, protein 26.4

Oregano Shrimp and Quinoa Salad

Preparation time: 5 minutes
Cooking time: 8 minutes
Servings: 4

Ingredients:

- 1 pound shrimp, peeled and deveined
- 1 cup quinoa, cooked
- Black pepper to the taste
- 1 tablespoon olive oil
- 1 tablespoon oregano, chopped
- 1 red onion, chopped
- Juice of 1 lemon

Directions:

1. Heat up a pan with the oil over medium-high heat, add the onion, stir and sauté for 2 minutes.
2. Add the shrimp, toss and cook for 5 minutes.
3. Add the rest of the ingredients, toss, divide everything into bowls and serve.

Nutrition: calories 336, fat 8.2, fiber 4.1, carbs 32.3, protein 32.3

Crab Salad

Preparation time: 10 minutes
Cooking time: 0 minutes
Servings: 4

Ingredients:
- 1 tablespoon olive oil
- 2 cups crab meat
- Black pepper to the taste
- 1 cup cherry tomatoes, halved
- 1 shallot, chopped
- 1 tablespoon lemon juice
- 1/3 cup cilantro, chopped

Directions:
1. In a bowl, combine the crab with the tomatoes and the other ingredients, toss and serve.

Nutrition: calories 54, fat 3.9, fiber 0.6, carbs 2.6, protein 2.3

Balsamic Scallops

Preparation time: 4 minutes
Cooking time: 6 minutes
Servings: 4

Ingredients:
- 12 ounces sea scallops
- 2 tablespoons olive oil
- 2 garlic cloves, minced
- 1 tablespoon balsamic vinegar
- 1 cup scallions, sliced
- 2 tablespoons cilantro, chopped

Directions:
1. Heat up a pan with the oil over medium heat, add the scallions and the garlic and sauté for 2 minutes.
2. Add the scallops and the other ingredients, cook them for 2 minutes on each side, divide between plates and serve.

Nutrition: calories 146, fat 7.7, fiber 0.7, carbs 4.4, protein 14.8

Creamy Flounder Mix

Preparation time: 10 minutes
Cooking time: 20 minutes
Servings: 4

Ingredients:
- 2 tablespoon olive oil
- 1 red onion, chopped
- Black pepper to the taste
- ½ cup low-sodium veggie stock
- 4 flounder fillets, boneless
- ½ cup coconut cream
- 1 tablespoon dill, chopped

Directions:
1. Heat up a pan with the oil over medium heat, add the onion, stir and sauté for 5 minutes.
2. Add the fish and cook it for 4 minutes on each side.
3. Add the rest of the ingredients, cook for 7 minutes more, divide between plates and serve.

Nutrition: calories 232, fat 12.3, fiber 4, carbs 8.7, protein 12

Spicy Salmon and Mango Mix

Preparation time: 5 minutes
Cooking time: 0 minutes
Servings: 4

Ingredients:

- 1 pound smoked salmon, boneless, skinless and flaked
- Black pepper to the taste
- 1 red onion, chopped
- 1 mango, peeled, seedless and chopped
- 2 jalapeno peppers, chopped
- ¼ cup parsley, chopped
- 3 tablespoons lime juice
- 1 tablespoon olive oil

Directions:

2. In a bowl, mix the salmon with the black pepper and the other ingredients, toss and serve.

Nutrition: calories 323, fat 14.2, fiber 4, carbs 8.5, protein 20.4

Dill Shrimp Mix

Preparation time: 5 minutes
Cooking time: 0 minutes
Servings: 4

Ingredients:
- 2 teaspoons lemon juice
- 1 tablespoon olive oil
- 1 tablespoon dill, chopped
- 1 pound shrimp, cooked, peeled and deveined
- Black pepper to the taste
- 1 cup radishes, cubed

Directions:
1. In a bowl, combine the shrimp with the lemon juice and the other ingredients, toss and serve.

Nutrition: calories 292, fat 13, fiber 4.4, carbs 8, protein 16.4

Salmon Pate

Preparation time: 4 minutes
Cooking time: 0 minutes
Servings: 6

Ingredients:

- 6 ounces smoked salmon, boneless, skinless and shredded
- 2 tablespoons non-fat yogurt
- 3 teaspoons lemon juice
- 2 spring onions, chopped
- 8 ounces low-fat cream cheese
- ¼ cup cilantro, chopped

Directions:

1. In a bowl, mix the salmon with the yogurt and the other ingredients, whisk and serve cold.

Nutrition: calories 272, fat 15.2, fiber 4.3, carbs 16.8, protein 9.9

Shrimp with Artichokes

Preparation time: 4 minutes
Cooking time: 8 minutes
Servings: 4

Ingredients:

- 2 green onions, chopped
- 1 cup canned artichokes, no-salt-added, drained and quartered
- 2 tablespoons cilantro, chopped
- 1 pound shrimp, peeled and deveined
- 1 cup cherry tomatoes, cubed
- 1 tablespoon olive oil
- 1 tablespoon balsamic vinegar
- A pinch of salt and black pepper

Directions:

1. Heat up a pan with the oil over medium heat, add the onions and the artichokes, toss and cook for 2 minutes.
2. Add the shrimp, toss and cook over medium heat for 6 minutes.
3. Divide everything into bowls and serve.

Nutrition: calories 260, fat 8.23, fiber 3.8, carbs 14.3, protein 12.4

Shrimp with Lemon Sauce

Preparation time: 5 minutes
Cooking time: 8 minutes
Servings: 4

Ingredients:

- 1 pound shrimp, peeled and deveined
- 2 tablespoons olive oil
- Zest of 1 lemon, grated
- Juice of ½ lemon
- 1 tablespoon chives, chopped

Directions:

1. Heat up a pan with the oil over medium-high heat, add the lemon zest, lemon juice and the cilantro, toss and cook for 2 minutes.
2. Add the shrimp, cook everything for 6 minutes more, divide between plates and serve.

Nutrition: calories 195, fat 8.9, fiber 0, carbs 1.8, protein 25.9

Tuna and Orange Mix

Preparation time: 5 minutes
Cooking time: 12 minutes
Servings: 4

Ingredients:
- 4 tuna fillets, boneless
- Black pepper to the taste
- 2 tablespoons olive oil
- 2 shallots, chopped
- 3 tablespoons orange juice
- 1 orange, peeled and cut into segments
- 1 tablespoon oregano, chopped

Directions:
1. Heat up a pan with the oil over medium-high heat, add the shallots, stir and sauté for 2 minutes.
2. Add the tuna and the other ingredients, cook everything for 10 minutes more, divide between plates and serve.

Nutrition: calories 457, fat 38.2, fiber 1.6, carbs 8.2, protein 21.8

Salmon Curry

Preparation time: 10 minutes
Cooking time: 20 minutes
Servings: 4

Ingredients:
- 1 pound salmon fillet, boneless and cubed
- 3 tablespoons red curry paste
- 1 red onion, chopped
- 1 teaspoon sweet paprika
- 1 cup coconut cream
- 1 tablespoon olive oil
- Black pepper to the taste
- ½ cup low-sodium chicken stock
- 3 tablespoons basil, chopped

Directions:
1. Heat up a pan with the oil over medium-high heat, add the onion, paprika and the curry paste, toss and cook for 5 minutes.
2. Add the salmon and the other ingredients, toss gently, cook over medium heat for 15 minutes, divide into bowls and serve.

Nutrition: calories 377, fat 28.3, fiber 2.1, carbs 8.5, protein 23.9

Salmon and Carrots Mix

Preparation time: 10 minutes
Cooking time: 15 minutes
Servings: 4

Ingredients:
- 4 salmon fillets, boneless
- 1 red onion, chopped
- 2 carrots, sliced
- 2 tablespoons olive oil
- 2 tablespoons balsamic vinegar
- Black pepper to the taste
- 2 tablespoons chives, chopped
- ¼ cup low-sodium veggie stock

Directions:
1. Heat up a pan with the oil over medium heat, add the onion and the carrots, toss and sauté for 5 minutes.
2. Add the salmon and the other ingredients, cook everything for 10 minutes more, divide between plates and serve.

Nutrition: calories 322, fat 18, fiber 1.4, carbs 6, protein 35.2

Shrimp and Pine Nuts Mix

Preparation time: 10 minutes
Cooking time: 10 minutes
Servings: 4

Ingredients:
- 1 pound shrimp, peeled and deveined
- 2 tablespoons pine nuts
- 1 tablespoon lime juice
- 2 tablespoons olive oil
- 3 garlic cloves, minced
- Black pepper to the taste
- 1 tablespoon thyme, chopped
- 2 tablespoons chives, finely chopped

Directions:
1. Heat up a pan with the oil over medium-high heat, add the garlic, thyme, pine nuts and lime juice, toss and cook for 3 minutes.
2. Add the shrimp, black pepper and the chives, toss, cook for 7 minutes more, divide between plates and serve.

Nutrition: calories 290, fat 13, fiber 4.5, carbs 13.9, protein 10

Chili Cod and Green Beans

Preparation time: 10 minutes
Cooking time: 14 minutes
Servings: 4

Ingredients:
- 4 cod fillets, boneless
- ½ pound green beans, trimmed and halved
- 1 tablespoon lime juice
- 1 tablespoon lime zest, grated
- 1 yellow onion, chopped
- 2 tablespoons olive oil
- 1 teaspoon cumin, ground
- 1 teaspoon chili powder
- ½ cup low-sodium veggie stock
- A pinch of salt and black pepper

Directions:
1. Heat up a pan with the oil over medium-high heat, add the onion, toss and cook for 2 minutes.
2. Add the fish and cook it for 3 minutes on each side.
3. Add the green beans and the rest of the ingredients, toss gently, cook for 7 minutes more, divide between plates and serve.

Nutrition: calories 220, fat 13, carbs 14.3, fiber 2.3, protein 12

Garlic Scallops

Preparation time: 5 minutes
Cooking time: 8 minutes
Servings: 4

Ingredients:
- 12 scallops
- 1 red onion, sliced
- 2 tablespoons olive oil
- ½ teaspoon garlic, minced
- 2 tablespoons lemon juice
- Black pepper to the taste
- 1 teaspoon balsamic vinegar

Directions:
1. Heat up a pan with the oil over medium heat, add the onion and the garlic and sauté for 2 minutes.
2. Add the scallops and the other ingredients, cook over medium heat for 6 minutes more, divide between plates and serve hot.

Nutrition: calories 259, fat 8, fiber 3, carbs 5.7, protein 7

Creamy Sea Bass Mix

Preparation time: 10 minutes
Cooking time: 14 minutes
Servings: 4

Ingredients:

- 4 sea bass fillets, boneless
- 1 cup coconut cream
- 1 yellow onion, chopped
- 1 tablespoon lime juice
- 2 tablespoons avocado oil
- 1 tablespoon parsley, chopped
- A pinch of black pepper

Directions:

1. Heat up a pan with the oil over medium heat, add the onion, toss and sauté for 2 minutes.
2. Add the fish and cook it for 4 minutes on each side.
3. Add the rest of the ingredients, cook everything for 4 minutes more, divide between plates and serve.

Nutrition: calories 283, fat 12.3, fiber 5, carbs 12.5, protein 8

Sea Bass and Mushrooms Mix

Preparation time: 10 minutes
Cooking time: 13 minutes
Servings: 4

Ingredients:
- 4 sea bass fillets, boneless
- 2 tablespoons olive oil
- Black pepper to the taste
- ½ cup white mushrooms, sliced
- 1 red onion, chopped
- 2 tablespoons balsamic vinegar
- 3 tablespoons cilantro, chopped

Directions:
1. Heat up a pan with the oil over medium-high heat, add the onion and the mushrooms, stir and cook for 5 minutes.
2. Add the fish and the other ingredients, cook for 4 minutes on each side, divide everything between plates and serve.

Nutrition: calories 280, fat 12.3, fiber 8, carbs 13.6, protein 14.3

Salmon Chowder

Preparation time: 5 minutes
Cooking time: 20 minutes
Servings: 4

Ingredients:

- 1 pound salmon fillets, boneless, skinless and cubed
- 1 cup yellow onion, chopped
- 2 tablespoons olive oil
- Black pepper to the taste
- 2 cups low-sodium veggie stock
- 1 and ½ cups tomatoes, chopped
- 1 tablespoon basil, chopped

Directions:

1. Heat up a pot with the oil over medium heat, add the onion, stir and sauté for 5 minutes.
2. Add the salmon and the other ingredients, bring to a simmer and cook over medium heat for 15 minutes.
3. Divide the chowder into bowls and serve.

Nutrition: calories 250, fat 12.2, fiber 5, carbs 8.5, protein 7

Nutmeg Shrimp

Preparation time: 3 minutes
Cooking time: 6 minutes
Servings: 4

Ingredients:

- 1 pound shrimp, peeled and deveined
- 2 tablespoons olive oil
- 1 tablespoon lemon juice
- 1 tablespoon nutmeg, ground
- Black pepper to the taste
- 1 tablespoon cilantro, chopped

Directions:

1. Heat up a pan with the oil over medium heat, add the shrimp, lemon juice and the other ingredients, toss, cook for 6 minutes, divide into bowls and serve.

Nutrition: calories 205, fat 9.6, fiber 0.4, carbs 2.7, protein 26

Shrimp and Berries Mix

Preparation time: 4 minutes
Cooking time: 6 minutes
Servings: 4

Ingredients:
- 1 pound shrimp, peeled and deveined
- ½ cup tomatoes, cubed
- 2 tablespoons olive oil
- 1 tablespoon balsamic vinegar
- ½ cup strawberries, chopped
- Black pepper to the taste

Directions:
1. Heat up a pan with the oil over medium heat, add the shrimp, toss and cook for 3 minutes.
2. Add the rest of the ingredients, toss, cook for 3-4 minutes more, divide into bowls and serve.

Nutrition: calories 205, fat 9, fiber 0.6, carbs 4, protein 26.2

Baked Lemony Trout

Preparation time: 10 minutes
Cooking time: 30 minutes
Servings: 4

Ingredients:
- 4 trout
- 1 tablespoon lemon zest, grated
- 2 tablespoons olive oil
- 2 tablespoons lemon juice
- A pinch of black pepper
- 2 tablespoons cilantro, chopped

Directions:
1. In a baking dish, combine the fish with the lemon zest and the other ingredients and rub.
2. Bake at 370 degrees F for 30 minutes, divide between plates and serve.

Nutrition: calories 264, fat 12.3, fiber 5, carbs 7, protein 11

Chives Scallops

Preparation time: 3 minutes
Cooking time: 4 minutes
Servings: 4

Ingredients:

- 12 scallops
- 2 tablespoons olive oil
- Black pepper to the taste
- 2 tablespoons chives, chopped
- 1 tablespoon sweet paprika

Directions:

1. Heat up a pan with the oil over medium heat, add the scallops, paprika and the other ingredients, and cook for 2 minutes on each side.
2. Divide between plates and serve with a side salad.

Nutrition: calories 215, fat 6, fiber 5, carbs 4.5, protein 11

Tuna Meatballs

Preparation time: 10 minutes
Cooking time: 30 minutes
Servings: 4

Ingredients:

- 2 tablespoons olive oil
- 1 pound tuna, skinless, boneless and minced
- 1 yellow onion, chopped
- ¼ cup chives, chopped
- 1 egg, whisked
- 1 tablespoon coconut flour
- A pinch of salt and black pepper

Directions:

1. In a bowl, mix the tuna with the onion and the other ingredients except the oil, stir well and shape medium meatballs out of this mix.
2. Arrange the meatballs on a baking sheet, grease them with the oil, introduce in the oven at 350 degrees F, cook for 30 minutes, divide between plates and serve.

Nutrition: calories 291, fat 14.3, fiber 5, carbs 12.4, protein 11

Salmon Pan

Preparation time: 10 minutes
Cooking time: 12 minutes
Servings: 4

Ingredients:

- 4 salmon fillets, boneless and roughly cubed
- 2 tablespoons olive oil
- 1 red bell pepper, cut into strips
- 1 zucchini, roughly cubed
- 1 eggplant, roughly cubed
- 1 tablespoon lemon juice
- 1 tablespoon dill, chopped
- ¼ cup low-sodium veggie stock
- 1 teaspoon garlic powder
- A pinch of black pepper

Directions:

1. Heat up a pan with oil over medium-high heat, add the bell pepper, zucchini and the eggplant, toss and sauté for 3 minutes.
2. Add the salmon and the other ingredients, toss gently, cook everything for 9 minutes more, divide between plates and serve.

Nutrition: calories 348, fat 18.4, fiber 5.3, carbs 11.9, protein 36.9

Mustard Cod Mix

Preparation time: 10 minutes
Cooking time: 25 minutes
Servings: 4

Ingredients:
- 4 cod fillets, skinless and boneless
- A pinch of black pepper
- 1 teaspoon ginger, grated
- 1 tablespoon mustard
- 2 tablespoons olive oil
- 1 teaspoon thyme, dried
- ¼ teaspoon cumin, ground
- 1 teaspoon turmeric powder
- ¼ cup cilantro, chopped
- 1 cup low-sodium veggie stock
- 3 garlic cloves, minced

Directions:
1. In a roasting pan, combine the cod with the black pepper, ginger and the other ingredients, toss gently and bake at 380 degrees F for 25 minutes.
2. Divide the mix between plates and serve.

Nutrition: calories 176, fat 9, fiber 1, carbs 3.7, protein 21.2

Shrimp and Asparagus Mix

Preparation time: 10 minutes
Cooking time: 14 minutes
Servings: 4

Ingredients:
- 1 asparagus bunch, halved
- 1 pound shrimp, peeled and deveined
- Black pepper to the taste
- 2 tablespoons olive oil
- 1 red onion, chopped
- 2 garlic cloves, minced
- 1 cup coconut cream

Directions:
1. Heat up a pan with the oil over medium heat, add the onion, garlic and the asparagus, toss and cook for 4 minutes.
2. Add the shrimp and the other ingredients, toss, simmer over medium heat for 10 minutes, divide everything into bowls and serve.

Nutrition: calories 225, fat 6, fiber 3.4, carbs 8.6, protein 8

Cod and Peas

Preparation time: 10 minutes
Cooking time: 20 minutes
Servings: 4

Ingredients:

- 1 yellow onion, chopped
- 2 tablespoons olive oil
- ½ cup low-sodium chicken stock
- 4 cod fillets, boneless, skinless
- Black pepper to the taste
- 1 cup snow peas

Directions:

1. Heat up a pot with the oil over medium heat, add the onion, stir and sauté fro 4 minutes.
2. Add the fish and cook it for 3 minutes on each side.
3. Add the snow peas and the other ingredients, cook everything for 10 minutes more, divide between plates and serve.

Nutrition: calories 240, fat 8.4, fiber 2.7, carbs 7.6, protein 14

Shrimp and Mussels Bowls

Preparation time: 5 minutes
Cooking time: 12 minutes
Servings: 4

Ingredients:
- 1 pound mussels, scrubbed
- ½ cup low-sodium chicken stock
- 1 pound shrimp, peeled and deveined
- 2 shallots, minced
- 1 cup cherry tomatoes, cubed
- 2 garlic cloves, minced
- 1 tablespoon olive oil
- Juice of 1 lemon

Directions:
1. Heat up a pan with the oil over medium heat, add the shallots and the garlic and sauté for 2 minutes.
2. Add the shrimp, mussels and the other ingredients, cook everything over medium heat for 10 minutes, divide into bowls and serve.

Nutrition: calories 240, fat 4.9, fiber 2.4, carbs 11.6, protein 8

Dash Diet Dessert Recipes

Mint Cream

Preparation time: 2 hours and 4 minutes

Cooking time: 0 minutes

Servings: 4

Ingredients:
- 4 cups non-fat yogurt
- 1 cup coconut cream
- 3 tablespoons stevia
- 2 teaspoons lime zest, grated
- 1 tablespoon mint, chopped

Directions:
1. In a blender, combine the cream with the yogurt and the other ingredients, pulse well, divide into cups and keep in the fridge for 2 hours before serving.

Nutrition: calories 512, fat 14.3, fiber 1.5, carbs 83.6, protein 12.1

Raspberries Pudding

Preparation time: 10 minutes
Cooking time: 24 minutes
Servings: 4

Ingredients:
- 1 cup raspberries
- 2 teaspoons coconut sugar
- 3 eggs, whisked
- 1 tablespoon avocado oil
- ½ cup almond milk
- ½ cup coconut flour
- ¼ cup non-fat yogurt

Directions:
1. In a bowl, combine the raspberries with the sugar and the other ingredients except the cooking spray and whisk well.
2. Grease a pudding pan with the cooking spray, add the raspberries mix, spread, bake in the oven at 400 degrees F for 24 minutes, divide between dessert plates and serve.

Nutrition: calories 215, fat 11.3, fiber 3.4, carbs 21.3, protein 6.7

Almond Bars

Preparation time: 10 minutes
Cooking time: 30 minutes
Servings: 4

Ingredients:

- 1 cup almonds, crushed
- 2 eggs, whisked
- ½ cup almond milk
- 1 teaspoon vanilla extract
- 2/3 cup coconut sugar
- 2 cups whole flour
- 1 teaspoon baking powder
- Cooking spray

Directions:

1. In a bowl, combine the almonds with the eggs and the other ingredients except the cooking spray and stir well.
2. Pour this into a square pan greased with cooking spray, spread well, bake in the oven for 30 minutes, cool down, cut into bars and serve.

Nutrition: calories 463, fat 22.5, fiber 11, carbs 54.4, protein 16.9

Baked Peaches Mix

Preparation time: 10 minutes
Cooking time: 30 minutes
Servings: 4

Ingredients:

- 4 peaches, stones removed and halved
- 1 tablespoon coconut sugar
- 1 teaspoon vanilla extract
- ¼ teaspoon cinnamon powder
- 1 tablespoon avocado oil

Directions:

1. In a baking pan, combine the peaches with the sugar and the other ingredients, bake at 375 degrees F for 30 minutes, cool down and serve.

Nutrition: calories 91, fat 0.8, fiber 2.5, carb 19.2, protein 1.7

Walnuts Cake

Preparation time: 10 minutes
Cooking time: 25 minutes
Servings: 8

Ingredients:
- 3 cups almond flour
- 1 cup coconut sugar
- 1 tablespoon vanilla extract
- ½ cup walnuts, chopped
- 2 teaspoons baking soda
- 2 cups coconut milk
- ½ cup coconut oil, melted

Directions:
1. In a bowl, combine the almond flour with the sugar and the other ingredients, whisk well, pour into a cake pan, spread, introduce in the oven at 370 degrees F, bake for 25 minutes.
2. Leave the cake to cool down, slice and serve.

Nutrition: calories 445, fat 10, fiber 6.5, carbs 31.4, protein 23.5

Apple Cake

Preparation time: 10 minutes
Cooking time: 30 minutes
Servings: 4

Ingredients:

- 2 cups almond flour
- 1 teaspoon baking soda
- 1 teaspoon baking powder
- ½ teaspoon cinnamon powder
- 2 tablespoons coconut sugar
- 1 cup almond milk
- 2 green apples, cored, peeled and chopped
- Cooking spray

Directions:

1. In a bowl, combine the flour with the baking soda, the apples and the other ingredients except the cooking spray, and whisk well.
2. Pour this into a cake pan greased with the cooking spray, spread well, introduce in the oven and bake at 360 degrees F for 30 minutes.
3. Cool the cake down, slice and serve.

Nutrition: calories 332, fat 22.4, fiber 91.6, carbs 22.2, protein 12.3

Cinnamon Cream

Preparation time: 2 hours
Cooking time: 10 minutes
Servings: 4

Ingredients:
- 1 cup non-fat almond milk
- 1 cup coconut cream
- 2 cups coconut sugar
- 2 tablespoons cinnamon powder
- 1 teaspoon vanilla extract

Directions:
1. Heat up a pan with the almond milk over medium heat, add the rest of the ingredients, whisk, and cook for 10 minutes more.
2. Divide the mix into bowls, cool down and keep in the fridge for 2 hours before serving.

Nutrition: calories 254, fat 7.5, fiber 5, carbs 16.4, protein 9.5

Creamy Strawberries Mix

Preparation time: 10 minutes
Cooking time: 0 minutes
Servings: 4

Ingredients:

- 1 teaspoon vanilla extract
- 2 cups strawberries, chopped
- 1 teaspoon coconut sugar
- 8 ounces non-fat yogurt

Directions:

1. In a bowl, combine the strawberries with the vanilla and the other ingredients, toss and serve cold.

Nutrition: calories 343, fat 13.4, fiber 6, carb 15.43, protein 5.5

Vanilla Pecan Brownies

Preparation time: 10 minutes
Cooking time: 25 minutes
Servings: 8

Ingredients:
- 1 cup pecans, chopped
- 3 tablespoons coconut sugar
- 2 tablespoons cocoa powder
- 3 eggs, whisked
- ¼ cup coconut oil, melted
- ½ teaspoon baking powder
- 2 teaspoons vanilla extract
- Cooking spray

Directions:
1. In your food processor, combine the pecans with the coconut sugar and the other ingredients except the cooking spray and pulse well.
2. Grease a square pan with cooking spray, add the brownies mix, spread, introduce in the oven, bake at 350 degrees F for 25 minutes, leave aside to cool down, slice and serve.

Nutrition: calories 370, fat 14.3, fiber 3, carbs 14.4, protein 5.6

Strawberries Cake

Preparation time: 10 minutes
Cooking time: 25 minutes
Servings: 6

Ingredients:
- 2 cups whole wheat flour
- 1 cup strawberries, chopped
- ½ teaspoon baking soda
- ½ cup coconut sugar
- ¾ cup coconut milk
- ¼ cup coconut oil, melted
- 2 eggs, whisked
- 1 teaspoon vanilla extract
- Cooking spray

Directions:
1. In a bowl, combine the flour with the strawberries and the other ingredients except the coking spray and whisk well.
2. Grease a cake pan with cooking spray, pour the cake mix, spread, bake in the oven at 350 degrees F for 25 minutes, cool down, slice and serve.

Nutrition: calories 465, fat 22.1, fiber 4, carbs 18.3, protein 13.4

Cocoa Pudding

Preparation time: 10 minutes
Cooking time: 10 minutes
Servings: 4

Ingredients:
- 2 tablespoons coconut sugar
- 3 tablespoons coconut flour
- 2 tablespoons cocoa powder
- 2 cups almond milk
- 2 eggs, whisked
- ½ teaspoon vanilla extract

Directions:
1. Put the milk in a pan, add the cocoa and the other ingredients, whisk, simmer over medium heat for 10 minutes, pour into small cups and serve cold.

Nutrition: calories 385, fat 31.7, fiber 5.7, carbs 21.6, protein 7.3

Nutmeg Vanilla Cream

Preparation time: 10 minutes
Cooking time: 0 minutes
Servings: 6

Ingredients:
- 3 cups non-fat milk
- 1 teaspoon nutmeg, ground
- 2 teaspoons vanilla extract
- 4 teaspoons coconut sugar
- 1 cup walnuts, chopped

Directions:
1. In a bowl, combine milk with the nutmeg and the other ingredients, whisk well, divide into small cups and serve cold.

Nutrition: calories 243, fat 12.4, fiber 1.5, carbs 21.1, protein 9.7

Avocado Cream

Preparation time: 1 hour and 10 minutes

Cooking time: 0 minutes
Servings: 4

Ingredients:
- 2 cups coconut cream
- 2 avocados, peeled, pitted and mashed
- 2 tablespoons coconut sugar
- 1 teaspoon vanilla extract

Directions:
1. In a blender, combine the cream with the avocados and the other ingredients, pulse well, divide into cups and keep in the fridge for 1 hour before serving.

Nutrition: calories 532, fat 48.2, fiber 9.4, carbs 24.9, protein 5.2

Raspberries Cream

Preparation time: 10 minutes
Cooking time: 25 minutes
Servings: 4

Ingredients:
- 2 tablespoons almond flour
- 1 cup coconut cream
- 3 cups raspberries
- 1 cup coconut sugar
- 8 ounces low-fat cream cheese

Directions:
1. In a bowl, the flour with the cream and the other ingredients, whisk, transfer to a round pan, cook at 360 degrees F for 25 minutes, divide into bowls and serve.

Nutrition: calories 429, fat 36.3, fiber 7.7, carbs 21.3, protein 7.8

Watermelon Salad

Preparation time: 4 minutes
Cooking time: 0 minutes
Servings: 4

Ingredients:

- 1 cup watermelon, peeled and cubed
- 2 apples, cored and cubed
- 1 tablespoon coconut cream
- 2 bananas, cut into chunks

Directions:

1. In a bowl, combine the watermelon with the apples and the other ingredients, toss and serve.

Nutrition: calories 131, fat 1.3, fiber 4.5, carbs 31.9, protein 1.3

Coconut Pears Mix

Preparation time: 10 minutes
Cooking time: 10 minutes
Servings: 4

Ingredients:
- 2 teaspoons lime juice
- ½ cup coconut cream
- ½ cup coconut, shredded
- 4 pears, cored and cubed
- 4 tablespoons coconut sugar

Directions:
1. In a pan, combine the pears with the lime juice and the other ingredients, stir, bring to a simmer over medium heat and cook for 10 minutes.
2. Divide into bowls and serve cold.

Nutrition: calories 320, fat 7.8, fiber 3, carbs 6.4, protein 4.7

Apples Compote

Preparation time: 10 minutes
Cooking time: 15 minutes
Servings: 4

Ingredients:

- 5 tablespoons coconut sugar
- 2 cups orange juice
- 4 apples, cored and cubed

Directions:

1. In a pot, combine apples with the sugar and the orange juice, toss, bring to a boil over medium heat, cook for 15 minutes, divide into bowls and serve cold.

Nutrition: calories 220, fat 5.2, fiber 3, carbs 5.6, protein 5.6

Apricots Stew

Preparation time: 10 minutes
Cooking time: 15 minutes
Servings: 4

Ingredients:
- 2 cups apricots, halved
- 2 cups water
- 2 tablespoons coconut sugar
- 2 tablespoons lemon juice

Directions:
1. In a pot, combine the apricots with the water and the other ingredients, toss, cook over medium heat for 15 minutes, divide into bowls and serve.

Nutrition: calories 260, fat 6.2, fiber 4.2, carbs 5.6, protein 6

Lemon Cantaloupe Mix

Preparation time: 10 minutes
Cooking time: 10 minutes
Servings: 4

Ingredients:
- 2 cups cantaloupe, peeled and roughly cubed
- 4 tablespoons coconut sugar
- 2 teaspoons vanilla extract
- 2 teaspoons lemon juice

Directions:
1. In a small pan, combine the cantaloupe with the sugar and the other ingredients, toss, heat up over medium heat, cook for about 10 minutes, divide into bowls and serve cold.

Nutrition: calories 140, fat 4, fiber 3.4, carbs 6.7, protein 5

Creamy Rhubarb Cream

Preparation time: 10 minutes
Cooking time: 14 minutes
Servings: 4

Ingredients:
- 1/3 cup low-fat cream cheese
- ½ cup coconut cream
- 2 pound rhubarb, roughly chopped
- 3 tablespoons coconut sugar

Directions:
1. In a blender, combine the cream cheese with the cream and the other ingredients and pulse well.
2. Divide into small cups, introduce in the oven and bake at 350 degrees F for 14 minutes.
3. Serve cold.

Nutrition: calories 360, fat 14.3, fiber 4.4, carbs 5.8, protein 5.2

Pineapple Bowls

Preparation time: 10 minutes
Cooking time: 0 minutes
Servings: 4

Ingredients:
- 3 cups pineapple, peeled and cubed
- 1 teaspoon chia seeds
- 1 cup coconut cream
- 1 teaspoon vanilla extract
- 1 tablespoon mint, chopped

Directions:
1. In a bowl, combine the pineapple with the cream and the other ingredients, toss, divide into smaller bowls and keep in the fridge for 10 minutes before serving.

Nutrition: calories 238, fat 16.6, fiber 5.6, carbs 22.8, protein 3.3

Blueberry Stew

Preparation time: 10 minutes
Cooking time: 10 minutes
Servings: 4

Ingredients:

- 2 tablespoons lemon juice
- 1 cup water
- 3 tablespoons coconut sugar
- 12 ounces blueberries

Directions:

1. In a pan, combine the blueberries with the sugar and the other ingredients, bring to a gentle simmer and cook over medium heat for 10 minutes.
2. Divide into bowls and serve.

Nutrition: calories 122, fat 0.4, fiber 2.1, carbs 26.7, protein 1.5

Lime Pudding

Preparation time: 10 minutes
Cooking time: 15 minutes
Servings: 4

Ingredients:
- 2 cups coconut cream
- Juice of 1 lime
- Zest of 1 lime, grated
- 3 tablespoons coconut oil, melted
- 1 egg, whisked
- 1 teaspoon baking powder

Directions:
1. In a bowl, combine the cream with the lime juice and the other ingredients and whisk well.
2. Divide into small ramekins, introduce in the oven and bake at 360 degrees F for 15 minutes.
3. Serve the pudding cold.

Nutrition: calories 385, fat 39.9, fiber 2.7, carbs 8.2, protein 4.2

Peach Cream

Preparation time: 10 minutes
Cooking time: 0 minutes
Servings: 4

Ingredients:

- 3 cups coconut cream
- 2 peaches, stones removed and chopped
- 1 teaspoon vanilla extract
- ½ cup almonds, chopped

Directions:

1. In a blender, combine the cream and the other ingredients, pulse well, divide into small bowls and serve cold.

Nutrition: calories 261, fat 13, fiber 5.6, carbs 7, protein 5.4

Cinnamon Plums Mix

Preparation time: 10 minutes
Cooking time: 15 minutes
Servings: 4

Ingredients:

- 1 pound plums, stones removed and halved
- 2 tablespoons coconut sugar
- ½ teaspoon cinnamon powder
- 1 cup water

Directions:

1. In a pan, combine the plums with the sugar and the other ingredients, bring to a simmer and cook over medium heat for 15 minutes.
2. Divide into bowls and serve cold.

Nutrition: calories 142, fat 4, fiber 2.4, carbs 14, protein 7

Chia and Vanilla Apples

Preparation time: 10 minutes
Cooking time: 10 minutes
Servings: 4

Ingredients:
- 2 cups apples, cored and cut into wedges
- 2 tablespoons chia seeds
- 1 teaspoon vanilla extract
- 2 cups naturally unsweetened apple juice

Directions:
1. In a small pot, combine the apples with the chia seeds and the other ingredients, toss, cook over medium heat for 10 minutes, divide into bowls and serve cold.

Nutrition: calories 172, fat 5.6, fiber 3.5, carbs 10, protein 4.4

Rice and Pears Pudding

Preparation time: 10 minutes
Cooking time: 25 minutes
Servings: 4

Ingredients:
- 6 cups water
- 1 cup coconut sugar
- 2 cups black rice
- 2 pears, cored and cubed
- 2 teaspoons cinnamon powder

Directions:
1. Put the water in a pan, heat it up over medium-high heat, add the rice, sugar and the other ingredients, stir, bring to a simmer, reduce heat to medium and cook for 25 minutes.
2. Divide into bowls and serve cold.

Nutrition: calories 290, fat 13.4, fiber 4, carbs 13.20, protein 6.7

Rhubarb Stew

Preparation time: 10 minutes
Cooking time: 15 minutes
Servings: 4

Ingredients:
- 2 cups rhubarb, roughly chopped
- 3 tablespoons coconut sugar
- 1 teaspoon almond extract
- 2 cups water

Directions:
1. In a pot, combine the rhubarb with the other ingredients, toss, bring to a boil over medium heat, cook for 15 minutes, divide into bowls and serve cold.

Nutrition: calories 142, fat 4.1, fiber 4.2, carbs 7, protein 4

Rhubarb Cream

Preparation time: 1 hour
Cooking time: 10 minutes
Servings: 4

Ingredients:

- 2 cups coconut cream
- 1 cup rhubarb, chopped
- 3 eggs, whisked
- 3 tablespoons coconut sugar
- 1 tablespoon lime juice

Directions:

1. In a small pan, combine the cream with the rhubarb and the other ingredients, whisk well, simmer over medium heat for 10 minutes, blend using an immersion blender, divide into bowls and keep in the fridge for 1 hour before serving.

Nutrition: calories 230, fat 8.4, fiber 2.4, carbs 7.8, protein 6

Blueberries Salad

Preparation time: 5 minutes
Cooking time: 0 minutes
Servings: 4

Ingredients:
- 2 cups blueberries
- 3 tablespoons mint, chopped
- 1 pear, cored and cubed
- 1 apple, core and cubed
- 1 tablespoon coconut sugar

Directions:
1. In a bowl, combine the blueberries with the mint and the other ingredients, toss and serve cold.

Nutrition: calories 150, fat 2.4, fiber 4, carbs 6.8, protein 6

Dates and Banana Cream

Preparation time: 5 minutes
Cooking time: 0 minutes
Servings: 4

Ingredients:

- 1 cup almond milk
- 1 banana, peeled and sliced
- 1 teaspoon vanilla extract
- ½ cup coconut cream
- dates, chopped

Directions:

1. In a blender, combine the dates with the banana and the other ingredients, pulse well, divide into small cups and serve cold.

Nutrition: calories 271, fat 21.6, fiber 3.8, carbs 21.2, protein 2.7

Plum Muffins

Preparation time: 10 minutes
Cooking time: 25 minutes
Servings: 12

Ingredients:
- 3 tablespoons coconut oil, melted
- ½ cup almond milk
- 4 eggs, whisked
- 1 teaspoon vanilla extract
- 1 cup almond flour
- 2 teaspoons cinnamon powder
- ½ teaspoon baking powder
- 1 cup plums, pitted and chopped

Directions:
1. In a bowl, combine the coconut oil with the almond milk and the other ingredients and whisk well.
2. Divide into a muffin pan, introduce in the oven at 350 degrees F and bake for 25 minutes.
3. Serve the muffins cold.

Nutrition: calories 270, fat 3.4, fiber 4.4, carbs 12, protein 5

Plums and Raisins Bowls

Preparation time: 10 minutes
Cooking time: 20 minutes
Servings: 4

Ingredients:
- ½ pound plums, pitted and halved
- 2 tablespoons coconut sugar
- 4 tablespoons raisins
- 1 teaspoon vanilla extract
- 1 cup coconut cream

Directions:
1. In a pan, combine the plums with the sugar and the other ingredients, bring to a simmer and cook over medium heat for 20 minutes.
2. Divide into bowls and serve.

Nutrition: calories 219, fat 14.4, fiber 1.8, carbs 21.1, protein 2.2

Sunflower Seed Bars

Preparation time: 10 minutes
Cooking time: 20 minutes
Servings: 6

Ingredients:
- 1 cup coconut flour
- ½ teaspoon baking soda
- 1 tablespoon flax seed
- 3 tablespoons almond milk
- 1 cup sunflower seeds
- 2 tablespoons coconut oil, melted
- 1 teaspoon vanilla extract

Directions:
1. In a bowl, mix the flour with the baking soda and the other ingredients, stir really well, spread on a baking sheet, press well, bake in the oven at 350 degrees F for 20 minutes, leave aside to cool down, cut into bars and serve.

Nutrition: calories 189, fat 12.6, fiber 9.2, carbs 15.7, protein 4.7

Blackberries and Cashews Bowls

Preparation time: 10 minutes

Cooking time: 0 minutes

Servings: 4

Ingredients:

- 1 cup cashews
- 2 cups blackberries
- ¾ cup coconut cream
- 1 teaspoon vanilla extract
- 1 tablespoon coconut sugar

Directions:

1.   In a bowl, combine the cashews with the berries and the other ingredients, toss, divide into small bowls and serve.

Nutrition: calories 230, fat 4, fiber 3.4, carbs 12.3, protein 8

Orange and Mandarins Bowls

Preparation time: 4 minutes
Cooking time: 8 minutes
Servings: 4

Ingredients:
- 4 oranges, peeled and cut into segments
- 2 mandarins, peeled and cut into segments
- Juice of 1 lime
- 2 tablespoons coconut sugar
- 1 cup water

Directions:
1. In a pan, combine the oranges with the mandarins and the other ingredients, bring to a simmer and cook over medium heat for 8 minutes.
2. Divide into bowls and serve cold.

Nutrition: calories 170, fat 2.3, fiber 2.3, carbs 11, protein 3.4

Pumpkin Cream

Preparation time: 2 hours
Cooking time: 0 minutes
Servings: 4

Ingredients:
- 2 cups coconut cream
- 1 cup pumpkin puree
- 14 ounces coconut cream
- 3 tablespoons coconut sugar

Directions:
1. In a bowl, combine the cream with the pumpkin puree and the other ingredients, whisk well, divide into small bowls and keep in the fridge for 2 hours before serving.

Nutrition: calories 350, fat 12.3, fiber 3, carbs 11.7, protein 6

Figs and Rhubarb Mix

Preparation time: 6 minutes
Cooking time: 14 minutes
Servings: 4

Ingredients:

- 2 tablespoons coconut oil, melted
- 1 cup rhubarb, roughly chopped
- 12 figs, halved
- ¼ cup coconut sugar
- 1 cup water

Directions:

1. Heat up a pan with the oil over medium heat, add the figs and the rest of the ingredients, toss, cook for 14 minutes, divide into small cups and serve cold.

Nutrition: calories 213, fat 7.4, fiber 6.1, carbs 39, protein 2.2

Spiced Banana

Preparation time: 4 minutes
Cooking time: 15 minutes
Servings: 4

Ingredients:
- 4 bananas, peeled and halved
- 1 teaspoon nutmeg, ground
- 1 teaspoon cinnamon powder
- Juice of 1 lime
- 4 tablespoons coconut sugar

Directions:
1. Arrange the bananas in a baking pan, add the nutmeg and the other ingredients, bake at 350 degrees F for 15 minutes.
2. Divide the baked bananas between plates and serve.

Nutrition: calories 206, fat 0.6, fiber 3.2, carbs 47.1, protein 2.4

Cocoa Smoothie

Preparation time: 5 minutes

Cooking time: 0 minutes

Servings: 2

Ingredients:

- 2 teaspoons cocoa powder
- 1 avocado, pitted, peeled and mashed
- 1 cup almond milk
- 1 cup coconut cream

Directions:

1. In your blender, combine the almond milk with the cream and the other ingredients, pulse well, divide in to cups and serve cold.

Nutrition: calories 155, fat 12.3, fiber 4, carbs 8.6, protein 5

Banana Bars

Preparation time: 30 minutes

Cooking time: 0 minutes

Servings: 4

Ingredients:

- 1 cup coconut oil, melted
- 2 bananas, peeled and chopped
- 1 avocado, peeled, pitted and mashed
- ½ cup coconut sugar
- ¼ cup lime juice
- 1 teaspoon lemon zest, grated
- Cooking spray

Directions:

1. In your food processor, mix the bananas with the oil and the other ingredients except the cooking spray and pulse well.
2. Grease a pan with the cooking spray, pour and spread the banana mix, spread, keep in the fridge for 30 minutes, cut into bars and serve.

Nutrition: calories 639, fat 64.6, fiber 4.9, carbs 20.5, protein 1.7

Green Tea and Dates Bars

Preparation time: 10 minutes
Cooking time: 30 minutes
Servings: 8

Ingredients:

- 2 tablespoons green tea powder
- 2 cups coconut milk, heated
- ½ cup coconut oil, melted
- 2 cups coconut sugar
- 4 eggs, whisked
- 2 teaspoons vanilla extract
- 3 cups almond flour
- 1 teaspoon baking soda
- 2 teaspoons baking powder

Directions:

1. In a bowl, combine the coconut milk with the green tea powder and the rest of the ingredients, stir well, pour into a square pan, spread, introduce in the oven, bake at 350 degrees F for 30 minutes, cool down, cut into bars and serve.

Nutrition: calories 560, fat 22.3, fiber 4, carbs 12.8, protein 22.1

Walnut Cream

Preparation time: 2 hours
Cooking time: 0 minutes
Servings: 4

Ingredients:
- 2 cups almond milk
- ½ cup coconut cream
- ½ cup walnuts, chopped
- 3 tablespoons coconut sugar
- 1 teaspoon vanilla extract

Directions:
1. In a bowl, combine the almond milk with the cream and the other ingredients, whisk well, divide into cups and keep in the fridge for 2 hours before serving.

Nutrition: calories 170, fat 12.4, fiber 3, carbs 12.8, protein 4

Lemon Cake

Preparation time: 10 minutes
Cooking time: 35 minutes
Servings: 6

Ingredients:
- 2 cups whole wheat flour
- 1 teaspoon baking powder
- 2 tablespoons coconut oil, melted
- 1 egg, whisked
- 3 tablespoons coconut sugar
- 1 cup almond milk
- Zest of 1 lemon, grated
- Juice of 1 lemon

Directions:
1. In a bowl, combine the flour with the oil and the other ingredients, whisk well, transfer this to a cake pan and bake at 360 degrees F for 35 minutes.
2. Slice and serve cold.

Nutrition: calories 222, fat 12.5, fiber 6.2, carbs 7, protein 17.4

Raisins Bars

Preparation time: 10 minutes
Cooking time: 25 minutes
Servings: 6

Ingredients:
- 1 teaspoon cinnamon powder
- 2 cups almond flour
- 1 teaspoon baking powder
- ½ teaspoon nutmeg, ground
- 1 cup coconut oil, melted
- 1 cup coconut sugar
- 1 egg, whisked
- 1 cup raisins

Directions:
1. In a bowl, combine the flour with the cinnamon and the other ingredients, stir well, spread on a lined baking sheet, introduce in the oven, bake at 380 degrees F for 25 minutes, cut into bars and serve cold.

Nutrition: calories 274, fat 12, fiber 5.2, carbs 14.5, protein 7

Nectarines Squares

Preparation time: 10 minutes
Cooking time: 20 minutes
Servings: 4

Ingredients:
- 3 nectarines, pitted and chopped
- 1 tablespoon coconut sugar
- ½ teaspoon baking soda
- 1 cup almond flour
- 4 tablespoons coconut oil, melted
- 2 tablespoons cocoa powder

Directions:
1. In a blender, combine the nectarines with the sugar and the rest of the ingredients, pulse well, pour into a lined square pan, spread, bake in the oven at 375 degrees F for 20 minutes, leave the mix aside to cool down a bit, cut into squares and serve.

Nutrition: calories 342, fat 14.4, fiber 7.6, carbs 12, protein 7.7

Grapes Stew

Preparation time: 10 minutes
Cooking time: 20 minutes
Servings: 4

Ingredients:
- 1 cup green grapes
- Juice of ½ lime
- 2 tablespoons coconut sugar
- 1 and ½ cups water
- 2 teaspoons cardamom powder

Directions:
1. Heat up a pan with the water medium heat, add the grapes and the other ingredients, bring to a simmer, cook for 20 minutes, divide into bowls and serve.

Nutrition: calories 384, fat 12.5, fiber 6.3, carbs 13.8, protein 5.6

Mandarin and Plums Cream

Preparation time: 10 minutes
Cooking time: 20 minutes
Servings: 4

Ingredients:
- 1 mandarin, peeled and chopped
- ½ pound plums, pitted and chopped
- 1 cup coconut cream
- Juice of 2 mandarins
- 2 tablespoons coconut sugar

Directions:
1. In a blender, combine the mandarin with the plums and the other ingredients, pulse well, divide into small ramekins, introduce in the oven, bake at 350 degrees F for 20 minutes, and serve cold.

Nutrition: calories 402, fat 18.2, fiber 2, carbs 22.2, protein 4.5

Cherry and Strawberries Cream

Preparation time: 10 minutes
Cooking time: 0 minutes
Servings: 6

Ingredients:

- 1 pound cherries, pitted
- 1 cup strawberries, chopped
- ¼ cup coconut sugar
- 2 cups coconut cream

Directions:

1. In a blender, combine the cherries with the other ingredients, pulse well, divide into bowls and serve cold.

Nutrition: calories 342, fat 22.1, fiber 5.6, carbs 8.4, protein 6.5

Cardamom Walnuts and Rice Pudding

Preparation time: 5 minutes
Cooking time: 40 minutes
Servings: 4

Ingredients:
- 1 cup basmati rice
- 3 cups almond milk
- 3 tablespoons coconut sugar
- ½ teaspoon cardamom powder
- ¼ cup walnuts, chopped

Directions:
1. In a pan, combine the rice with the milk and the other ingredients, stir, cook for 40 minutes over medium heat, divide into bowls and serve cold.

Nutrition: calories 703, fat 47.9, fiber 5.2, carbs 62.1, protein 10.1

Pears Bread

Preparation time: 10 minutes
Cooking time: 30 minutes
Servings: 4

Ingredients:
- 2 cups pears, cored and cubed
- 1 cup coconut sugar
- 2 eggs, whisked
- 2 cups almond flour
- 1 tablespoon baking powder
- 1 tablespoon coconut oil, melted

Directions:
1. In a bowl, mix the pears with the sugar and the other ingredients, whisk, pour into a loaf pan, introduce in the oven and bake at 350 degrees F for 30 minutes.
2. Slice and serve cold.

Nutrition: calories 380, fat 16.7, fiber 5, carbs 17.5, protein 5.6

Rice and Cherries Pudding

Preparation time: 10 minutes
Cooking time: 25 minutes
Servings: 4

Ingredients:

- 1 tablespoon coconut oil, melted
- 1 cup white rice
- 3 cups almond milk
- ½ cup cherries, pitted and halved
- 3 tablespoons coconut sugar
- 1 teaspoon cinnamon powder
- 1 teaspoon vanilla extract

Directions:

1. In a pan, combine the oil with the rice and the other ingredients, stir, bring to a simmer, cook for 25 minutes over medium heat, divide into bowls and serve cold.

Nutrition: calories 292, fat 12.4, fiber 5.6, carbs 8, protein 7

Watermelon Stew

Preparation time: 5 minutes
Cooking time: 8 minutes
Servings: 4

Ingredients:

- Juice of 1 lime
- 1 teaspoon lime zest, grated
- 1 and ½ cup coconut sugar
- 4 cups watermelon, peeled and cut into large chunks
- 1 and ½ cups water

Directions:

1. In a pan, combine the watermelon with the lime zest, and the other ingredients, toss, bring to a simmer over medium heat, cook for 8 minutes, divide into bowls and serve cold.

Nutrition:: calories 233, fat 0.2, fiber 0.7, carbs 61.5, protein 0.9

Ginger Pudding

Preparation time: 1 hour
Cooking time: 0 minutes
Servings: 4

Ingredients:
- 2 cups almond milk
- ½ cup coconut cream
- 2 tablespoons coconut sugar
- 1 tablespoon ginger, grated
- ¼ cup chia seeds

Directions:
1. In a bowl, combine the milk with the cream and the other ingredients, whisk well, divide into small cups and keep them in the fridge for 1 hour before serving.

Nutrition: calories 345, fat 17, fiber 4.7, carbs 11.5, protein 6.9

Cashew Cream

Preparation time: 2 hours
Cooking time: 0 minutes
Servings: 4

Ingredients:

- 1 cup cashews, chopped
- 2 tablespoons coconut oil, melted
- 2 tablespoons coconut oil, melted
- 1 cup coconut cream
- tablespoons lemon juice
- 1 tablespoons coconut sugar

Directions:

1. In a blender, combine the cashews with the coconut oil and the other ingredients, pulse well, divide into small cups and keep in the fridge for 2 hours before serving.

Nutrition: calories 480, fat 43.9, fiber 2.4, carbs 19.7, protein 7

Hemp Cookies

Preparation time: 30 minutes
Cooking time: 0 minutes
Servings: 6

Ingredients:
- 1 cup almonds, soaked overnight and drained
- 2 tablespoons cocoa powder
- 1 tablespoon coconut sugar
- ½ cup hemp seeds
- ¼ cup coconut, shredded
- ½ cup water

Directions:
1. In your food processor, combine the almonds with the cocoa powder and the other ingredients, pulse well, press this on a lined baking sheet, keep in the fridge for 30 minutes, slice and serve.

Nutrition: calories 270, fat 12.6, fiber 3, carbs 7.7, protein 7

Almonds and Pomegranate Bowls

Preparation time: 2 hours
Cooking time: 0 minutes
Servings: 4

Ingredients:
- ½ cup coconut cream
- 1 teaspoon vanilla extract
- 1 cup almonds, chopped
- 1 cup pomegranate seeds
- 1 tablespoon coconut sugar

Directions:
1. In a bowl, combine the almonds with the cream and the other ingredients, toss, divide into small bowls and serve.

Nutrition: calories 258, fat 19, fiber 3.9, carbs 17.6, protein 6.2

CPSIA information can be obtained
at www.ICGtesting.com
Printed in the USA
BVHW070053220722
642761BV00008B/698

9 781837 891047